THE BOOK OF HEALTH

Susan Stockton

Illustrations by Penny Jensen

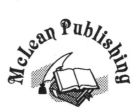

McLean Publishing

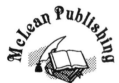
McLean Publishing
8709 Somersworth Place
Tampa, Florida 33634

First Printing December 1990
Second Printing January 1991
Third Printing June 1992
Fourth Printing November 1993

ISBN 0-9628770-0-X

To my dear friend, student and teacher, Bryant Gardner whose advice, patience, help and word processor made this book possible!

To my Health Care Alternatives students who have provided the impetus and a good deal of the information that has gone into this project.

I also want to thank Susan McLean for her patient, careful and caring execution of this project.

A special thank you also to Pepito Valdes for taking time to contribute his photographic skills.

TABLE OF CONTENTS

CONTENTS

CONTENTS

INTRODUCTION

This book deals with health and the components of a healthy lifestyle. Although a good portion deals with diet, the aim is not to dictate menus, but rather to instruct in basic principles of nutrition so that intelligent choices can be made regarding food. There will, of course, be some foods to avoid and their avoidance will require discipline. Such discipline is to be viewed not as a restriction or deprivation however, but rather as a tool to a fuller and more abundant life, for any discipline which leads to wellness and vitality becomes a joy to follow and not a burden.

'Lifestyle' encompasses much more than diet. It includes all of our choices and activities which reflect basic attitudes and values. Factors motivating lifestyle choices are both personal and interpersonal. On a personal level, a prime determining factor is willingness to take responsibility for one's own health. Interpersonal aspects emerge in terms of degree of need to conform.

The health conscious individual in today's society must have achieved a degree of independence and self-confidence sufficient to empower him* to take responsibility for his health without depending upon an authority figure to make his decisions for him. He must have the insight and intelligence to realize that every choice he makes in his daily life either builds health or does not. And, of course, he must have **information**, knowledge upon which to base his choices. It is the better part of wisdom to seek counsel with professionals in the field to obtain advice and recommendations, but we must ultimately develop the competence and confidence to make our own decisions. This means taking a stand on what we believe. In weighing opinion on controversial health matters, we must consider the source of the information, as well as the probable motivation underlying the conclusion. Could the researcher possibly have a *vested interest* in obtaining a certain outcome that may bias his findings? This is an important question to consider. When nutritional research is conducted by a manufacturer of a certain food product, it is highly likely that the results of his study will emphasize the beneficial aspects of his product and not represent an objective, unbiased conclusion. Much nutritional research today *is* conducted by food manufacturers and much of the 'education' received by the general public is provided by commercial advertising. And the medical doctor is getting a good deal of *his* continuing education from the detail men from the pharmaceutical companies (who also sell nutritional supplements), another case of vested interest.

Conforming behaviors in today's fast food, high stress society are not an asset as far as health matters go, for the lifestyle of the masses has been a significant factor in the escalation of degenerative disease since the turn of the century. This is a premise which is more fully developed throughout the text.

As the 'New Age', symbolized by the air sign, Aquarius, progresses, it brings into our consciousness the potential of air waves ($\approx$) or electricity as a major healing modality. Our awareness of the electrical nature of the body comes also into manifestation in this age. And the Aquarian qualities of intelligence, independent thinking, progressive outlook and love of freedom serve the New Age time traveler well in his quest for health on this polluted planet.

---

* The words 'him' and 'he' are used throughout this book in place of him/her and he/she for convenience only. They are intended to encompass the female as well as the male gender.

ONE

OVERCONSUMPTION MALNUTRITION

Americans are proud. We like to think of our nation as the greatest in the world - the wealthiest, the strongest, the healthiest. We certainly have the material wealth and, if it could buy health, perhaps we'd have that too. It's not that we don't try. We spend in the neighborhood of half a trillion dollars per year on "health care", more than any other nation in the world. And yet, in terms of longevity, we fare very poorly, the mortality rate of our females ranking 14th in the world, males 19th.

In 1900 America **was** the healthiest nation in the world. By 1920 we dropped down to the #2 spot (of 93 civilized nations) and by 1978 we ranked #79. Each year we have dropped down by about 2 places. So, where have we gone wrong, why this deplorable state of health? Why this rampant onslaught of degenerative disease where approximately 120,000 people die **each month** of cancer, heart disease, arthritis, diabetes, etc. (the bomb we dropped on Hiroshima only killed 70,000)? As things stand now, one out of every three people will develop cancer and one of two of those will die from it. One of two will develop heart disease. Too few people are dying these days of "natural causes" to be calculated in mortality statistics. It's degenerative disease that is claiming so many lives. And not just among the elderly. Cancer is now the leading cause of childhood death, barring accidents.

What we'd like to begin looking at in the remaining pages of this chapter are the causes of this escalation in degenerative disease. As a working premise we'd like to suggest that a basic cause for this increase is the prevalence of a condition which has been referred to as overconsumption malnutrition. OVER-CONSUMPTION MALNUTRITION: The American plague. What is it? It is, as its name implies, a condition wherein the body is malnourished, while simultaneously being overfed. We tend to think of malnourishment as resulting from **under**eating, but, in actuality, it is a consequence of taking too little **nourishment** into the system. The amount of nourishment a meal provides is not measured by the quantity of food, but rather by the **quality** of the food. We can (and do) eat tremendous quantities of food and still be malnourished (and therefore still hungry) because the quality of the food is substandard. Are we suggesting that the Standard American Diet (SAD) may be substandard? Yes, we are. And moreover, we maintain that the SAD, composed of processed, refined, preserved, irradiated, enriched and otherwise devitalized food-like substances, is a root cause of the increase in degenerative diseases in our culture. And so, we postulate a cause-effect relationship that looks like this:

Intake of devitalized food
▼
Condition of overconsumption malnutrition
▼
Increase in degenerative disease

Let's look now at some of the factors responsible for this situation. On the top of the list, we would place:

THE ECONOMIC EXPEDIENCY OF MARKETING DEVITALIZED FOODS

Under this heading we include the practices of **refining, enriching** and **preserving** foods. The dictionary defines "refined" as (1) free from coarseness or vulgarity (2) free of impurities (3) precise to a fine degree; subtle, exact. All of these definitions have positive connotations which might lead one to believe that the refining process is a beneficial one. It is not. The food processors give a whole new dimension to the meaning of the word. The same may be said of "enriched". The name implies that the product has more or better ingredients than its unenriched counterpart. Not so again. These are misleading terms. Any refined food product has been altered from its natural state, subjected to a process that destroys much of its nutritional value. UNrefined is natural. Refined is not.

In 1862 machinery was invented which permitted milling of grains, giving them a lighter color, a finer texture - and a poorer nutrient content. The refining of grains involves the removal and disposal of their outer husks where most of the nutrients are concentrated. Wheat germ and bran, rice polish - these are removed during the milling process. Elimination of these nutritious parts of the grain from our diet has resulted in a widespread deficiency of B vitamins (see chapter 8). Other vitamins and minerals, as well as fiber are likewise lost. And the devitalized "enriched" product, such as white flour, acts quite literally like paste in the intestines (flour + water = paste. Remember that from grammar school?). Lately, Americans have developed a fiber consciousness of sorts and consequently have purchased bran by the pound. The food processor is more than willing to increase his profits by packaging and marketing that portion of the grain that was formerly shipped off for animal feed. He profits twice, for the uninformed consumer purchases both the enriched grain product **and** a bag of bran to further enrich it, unaware that the grain in its natural state contained the bran until it was refined. Some of us are getting wise and purchasing the whole grain product instead. Some of us have even learned that fiber isn't found only in packages in grocery stores and in grains, but richly abounds in fruits and vegetables.

During World War I the milling of grains was forbidden in Denmark due to economic cutbacks. It is interesting to note that the death rate subsequently fell 34%...during the **war** years! The incidence of cancer, kidney disease and diabetes (our top three degenerative diseases) also dropped markedly. Much the same thing happened in England during World War II when grains were only slightly milled.

White flour products are examples of refined grains. White rice is another example. When white rice took the world by storm and replaced its longer cooking brown counterpart, there ensued the development of a dreaded disease named beri-beri. About this time in history, the germ theory had gained wide spread acceptance and scientists were being offered incentives to find the "germ" responsible for causing the disease. They never did find it because beri-beri is not caused by a germ, but rather by a nutritional deficiency. This was discovered accidently when sick animals were fed brown rice rejected for human consumption and became well. Thiamine or vitamin B1 is a component of the husk of brown rice. It is essential for the health of the nervous system. When the husks of the rice are discarded during the refining process so is the B1, along with other B vitamins.

As time passed, it became embarrassingly obvious that the refining process destroyed vital nutrients. Enter the **enriching** process in 1941. Ever see one of those labels that reads something like "ENRICHED with vitamin B1, B2, niacin and iron?" Wow! - this means that three B vitamins and one mineral (in their synthetic form) are added to a grain product that, before it was 'refined', contained those nutrients in their natural form plus many, many more. So - the "enriching" process puts back a little - a very little - of what the refining process took out! The grain product is then about as enriched as you would be if someone stole $5000 from you and gave you back $100. We can all think of more appropriate and accurate names than "enriched" for this process, but they wouldn't make for sound marketing strategy! Remember - anything that's enriched has first been impoverished.

There are currently some 3000 additives in our food supply. This amounts to approximately ten pounds of food additives - emulsifiers, stabilizers, thickeners, flavoring and coloring agents, preservatives, etc. - consumed per person per year. Extending shelf life is the major goal of the food preservatives. And indeed shelf life is extended, for, as Adelle Davis pointed out in the 60's, the preserved food "can't even support the health of bacteria, molds, weevils" (Let's Eat Right To Keep Fit). Obviously it cannot support human health either.

The following exposé about additives used in ice cream appeared in the June 1958 edition of the magazine, Nature's Path:

In the old days when ice cream was made of whole eggs, milk and sugar and laboriously cranked out in the old home freezer, a serving of ice cream was only an occasional family treat which didn't do much harm. Today, in this mass-producing, synthetic age, it is another matter entirely. Today you may be "treating" your family to POISON.

Ice cream manufacturers are not required by law to list the additives used in the manufacture of their product. Consequently, today most ice creams are synthetic from start to finish. Analysis has shown the following:

DIETHYL GLUCOL - a cheap chemical used as an emulsifier instead of eggs is the same chemical used in anti-freeze and in paint removers.

PIPERONAL - used in place of vanilla. This is a chemical used to kill lice.

ALDEHYDE C 17 - used to flavor cherry ice cream. It is an in-flammable liquid which is also used in aniline dyes, plastic and rubber.

ETHYL ACETATE - used to give ice cream a pineapple flavor. It is also used as a cleaner for leather and textiles and its vapors have been known to cause chronic lung, liver and heart damage.

BUTYRALDEHYDE - used in nut flavored ice cream. It's one of the ingredients in rubber cement.

AMYL ACETATE - used for its banana flavor. It's also used as an oil paint solvent.

BENZYL ACETATE - used for its strawberry flavor. It's a nitrate solvent.

The next time you're tempted by a luscious looking banana split sundae, think of it as a mixture of anti-freeze, oil paint, nitrate solvent, and lice killer and you won't find it so appetizing!

Aside from the physical effects of food additives, they can affect us on an emotional level as well. Dr. Benjamin Feingold brought to the attention of the American public the link between food additives and hyperactive behavior in children and demonstrated how the condition could be brought under control through diet, without the use of drugs.

Too few of us bother to read ingredients on labels. There's an art to it. Or perhaps it's more of a science. A background in chemistry would certainly be helpful in deciphering many a label, replete as they tend to be with chemical jargon. A good rule of thumb is this: If the list of ingredients is lengthy and the words hard to pronounce **don't buy it**. It's useful to know that ingredients are listed in descending order in terms of quantity present in the food. For example, if sugar is the #1 ingredient (as it so often is), there's more of it than anything else in the food. If the last ingredient listed is salt, there's less salt (though there still may be a considerable amount of it) than any other ingredient.

Lest we worry overmuch about the possible damage caused by the 3000 or so additives in our food supply, the government offers new hope, an alternative to chemical preservatives or at least a method that will help decrease their use and still prolong shelf life:

FOOD IRRADIATION

Food irradiation is a process wherein food items ride on a conveyor belt into a chamber where they will be zapped with gamma rays, a form of ionizing radiation, for the purpose of preserving them.

It was in the 1930's that the food irradiation process was first patented by French scientists. In the early 60's it was approved by the FDA for use on wheat and potatoes. It was not taken too seriously, however, at that time, as cheaper chemical methods of preservation were preferred. However, in 1984 a fresh look was taken at the process after EDB (ethylene dibromide), a widely used chemical, was banned. By 7/85 the irradiation of pork was approved at a rate two times higher than for wheat. In 4/86 the irradiation of fruits and vegetables at the same dose as pork was approved. That dose is up to 100,000 RADS (Radiation Absorbed Doses). At the same time, the irradiation of herbs and spices was approved at a rate 60 times higher than previous levels or 3 million RADS. 3 million RADS is the equivalent of **2 million chest x-rays**!

Irradiated food is not necessarily labeled, at least not in the sense that it is stamped with the word "irradiated". The display of the radura symbol has been proposed as a substitute for use of the word "irradiated". This stylized flower in itself gives no suggestion that the food has been penetrated with gamma rays, infused with nuclear waste. Opponents of food irradiation suggest that a skull & cross bones might be a more appropriate symbol! Even the radura would appear only when the entire food has been irradiated. Exempt from the requirement of bearing the radura symbol or other markings indicating irradiation are processed & packaged foods which may have irradiated ingredients in them. Also exempt are restaurant and institutional foods.

As of this writing (5/90), Food and Water, Inc. informs

us that "The FDA decided that all whole foods which have been irradiated must be labeled. However, spices, ingredients and foods which contain irradiated ingredients do not require a label. This decision has no definite time limit."

Australia, New Zealand, Sweden and West Germany have banned food irradiation. So have New Jersey, New York and Maine to date.

While the federal government claims the absolute safety of the food irradiation process, the fact of the matter is that the FDA approval of the process was not based on tests demonstrating its safety, but rather upon the theoretical estimate of the number of unique radiolytic products (URP's) in which they are likely to result. To understand what this means, we have to first understand that gamma rays, with their ionizing effect, have the ability to knock electrons out of atoms. Ionizing radiation gives rise to the creation of free radicals, renegade chemical fragments which have been demonstrated to play a significant role in the aging and degenerative disease processes. The free radical is a molecule with an unpaired electron, of either a positive or negative charge. A URP is formed when two of these chemical fragments of unlike charges unite. A myriad of possible combinations is created, with the possibility of some of the newly created URP's being carcinogenic.

As far as studies go, the first research done in this country was in the 50s on canned bacon in the Army. The 1963 FDA clearance of the use of the irradiated product was withdrawn in 1968 due to the discovery that the research was flawed. Much of the research supporting food irradiation was carried out by Industrial Biotest Limited. In 1983 three of their officials were convicted in federal court for fraudulent research for government and industry. And yet the federal government assures us that studies indicated that the process is safe. What studies? Surely not the ones conducted in 1975 on Indian children who showed blood changes similar to leukemia three weeks after consuming freshly irradiated wheat? Surely not those studies that prompted Germany and Great Britain to ban food irradiation? Harvey Diamond tells us that "an internal 1982 FDA audit showed that only 1% of 413 studies conducted over 30 years appeared to support safety (of the process)" (Fit for Life II, p.126).

Ill effects cited by German scientists included mutations, decreased growth rate, reduced resistance to disease, changes in organ weight and development of tumors. Kidney damage has also resulted from the irradiation process. It should also be pointed out that nutrients are destroyed or modified by the ionizing effect of radiation. An estimated 20-80% of vitamins A, B, C, E, and K and the essential fatty acids are thus affected. With this kind of nutrient loss upon irradiation, further loss during storage and even further nutrient depletion with cooking, with what are we left? We're left with food that is even more devitalized than it now is.

Proponents of food irradiation point out that it destroys bacteria. It should be noted, however, that, even if bacteria are killed, toxins that have been created by the bacteria at earlier stages of contamination are not removed. It is observed also that irradiation at approved levels slows the ripening of fruits and vegetables, but is not high enough to destroy such microorganisms as botulism. The smell however is eradicated, increasing the danger of consumption of contaminated food. Another concern is the probable proliferation of toxic, radiation-resistant micro-organisms.

The government has plans for building 1000 food irradiation plants, each using from 1-10 million curies of radioactive material. This is more than 1000 times the amount released by a 20 kiloton nuclear bomb. The environmental and safety hazards posed by the operation of such plants is a further concern. And it is not exactly reassuring that Dr. Martin Welt was appointed by the Department of Energy as advisor to the Advisory Committee to plan six DOE funded demonstration irradiation plants. Dr. Welt was founder and president of Radiation Technology, Inc. which was "cited 32 times for various violations, including throwing radioactive garbage out with the regular trash." In 1977 one worker in that plant received a near lethal dosage of radiation when the device that prevents people from entering the irradiation cell during operation (the interlock safety device) was bypassed by order of Dr. Welt, who later gave false information on the incident to the Nuclear Regulatory Commission (Food Irradiation - Who Wants It?, page 68).

If food irradiation is so bad, who wants it and why? Harvey Diamond seems to hit the nail on the head with his statement: "the purpose of irradiating food is to rid the Department of Energy of its nuclear waste problem and to make a profit for the food industry at the same time" (Fit for Life II, p. 128). There are two radioactive isotopes which are typically used in the food irradiation process - cobalt 60 and cesium 137. They are nuclear waste products. Cesium 137 is a byproduct of plutonium extraction. The U.S. military has an avid interest in plutonium, as it is used in the production of some 1800 nuclear warheads per year in this country. However, in 1982 Congress placed a ban on the reprocessing of commercial wastes. This prohibited the military from retrieving the plutonium. Now with a "viable"(?) use found for the cesium 137 (putting it in our food), the military can once again get at the plutonium. So, the military profits, the food industry profits, but what of the planet as a whole and the life it supports? Cobalt 60 is hazardous to all who come into contact with it for 50 - 100 years. Cesium 137 remains hazardous for 300 - 600 years. It is also fully water soluble. That means that if it leaches into underground water, it will be impossible to retrieve.

Given the available information, we concur with Mr. Diamond that "food irradiation has **nothing** to do with shelf life and killing bacteria. It has to do with pluto-

nium and nuclear warheads" (<u>Fit for Life II</u>, p. 130).
It is plain to see, on the basis of the foregoing data, how
vested financial interest within the food industry, with
its practices of "refinement", "enrichment", chemical
preservation and now food irradiation, is making a
huge contribution to the devitalization and contamination of our food supply and thus to the condition of
overconsumption malnutrition. A question that logi-
cally ensues is, "how can this be happening?", how can
we **allow** this to happen? Unfortunately, due largely
to overwhelmingly successful advertising efforts,
Americans are not only allowing, but are now **demanding** the production and delivery of fast foods,
junk foods, non-food foods. A major reason for this is
seen as:

LACK OF EDUCATION

We speak here not only of the lack of education of the
general public, but also a deficiency of education
within the medical profession. Only 1/3 of our 127
medical schools offer courses in nutrition and only
half of those make enrollment in them mandatory.
What little nutrition education that is offered, both in
medical schools and in other institutions of learning, is
based, for the most part, on the well known "Four
Food Groups": meat, dairy products, cereal grains
and fruits/vegetables. The origin of the Four Food
Groups lies not in the scientific realm, but once again
in the domain of vested interest within the food industry. The idea of the Four Food Groups was introduced by the Kellogg people (of corn flake fame) in
conjunction with the dairy industry. The meat people
later joined them. It has been suggested that the Four
Food Groups might more accurately be referred to as
the Four Food **Lobbies**!

As the late Dr. Robert Mendelsohn, M.D. repeatedly
pointed out, the "Church of Modern Medicine" is the
religion of the masses in the U.S. The word "doctor"
is synonymous with **medical** doctor in the minds of
most. We have been very thoroughly indoctrinated to

believe that allopathic medicine (the chemically oriented kind that we know and love) is the **only valid system** of health care. We're led to believe that other systems are "unscientific quackery" and we're cautioned to "Beware of the Health Hucksters" (title of a recent Reader's Digest article) who offer "dangerous" alternatives. One cannot help but wonder what is endangered - the health of the people or the reign of the medical monopoly?

The truth of the matter is that, despite AMA propaganda, the **medical** doctor is **not** the only type of physician practicing in this country, nor is he the only type of **qualified, competent, licensed** physician. Three other types of physicians are trained and licensed in the U.S. at present: chiropractors (D.C.s), osteopaths (D.O.s) and naturopaths (N.D.s). Let's take a look at each of these professions:

CHIROPRACTIC

Chiropractic, as an organized system of health care, was developed by D.D. Palmer in 1895. It is based on the theory that disease is due primarily to impingement of nerves. As the spinal chart (page 15) shows, the spine is divided into segments: cervical (neck), thoracic (mid back) and lumbar (lower back). Between each vertebra or large bone in these segments, spinal nerves are interlaced. These nerves all lead to specific areas of the body. For example, note that T-10 (the tenth thoracic vertebra) leads to the kidneys. If a patient is suffering from a kidney disorder, the doctor of chiropractic would most certainly be interested in the positioning of T-10. If it is **subluxated** or misaligned, it would be exerting pressure or impinging upon the tenth thoracic nerve which supplies nerve energy to the kidneys. That organ then would be hampered in its ability to receive nerve impulses. Circulation too would be impaired, with lack of nutrients and oxygen to the kidney area. By re-seating the vertebrae into their correct positions (at the level of T-10 and elsewhere), proper nerve supply and circu-

SPINAL

CHART

	Vertebrae	Areas
ATLAS		
AXIS		
CERVICAL SPINE	1C	Blood supply to the head, pituitary gland, scalp, bones of the face, brain, inner and middle ear, sympathetic nervous system.
	2C	Eyes, optic nerves, auditory nerves, sinuses, mastoid bones, tongue, forehead.
1st THORACIC	3C	Cheeks, outer ear, face bones, teeth, trifacial nerve.
	4C	Nose, lips, mouth, eustachian tube.
	5C	Vocal cords, neck glands, pharynx.
	6C	Neck muscles, shoulders, tonsils.
	7C	Thyroid gland, bursae in the shoulders, elbows.
THORACIC SPINE	1T	Arms from the elbows down, including hands, wrists, and fingers, esophagus and trachea.
	2T	Heart, including its valves and covering, coronary arteries.
	3T	Lungs, bronchial tubes, pleura, chest, breast.
	4T	Gall bladder, common duct.
	5T	Liver, solar plexus, circulation (general).
	6T	Stomach.
	7T	Pancreas, duodenum.
	8T	Spleen.
	9T	Adrenal and supra-renal glands.
1st LUMBAR	10T	Kidneys.
	11T	Kidney, ureters.
	12T	Small intestines, lymph circulation.
LUMBAR SPINE	1L	Large intestines, inguinal rings.
	2L	Appendix, abdomen, upper leg.
	3L	Sex organs, uterus, bladder, knees.
SACRUM	4L	Prostate gland, muscles of the lower back, sciatic nerve.
	5L	Lower legs, ankles, feet.
	SACRUM	Hip bones, buttocks.
COCCYX	COCCYX	Rectum, anus.

lation are restored to the kidneys and other organs and the body then has the energy available to it to mobilize its own healing resources. The re-seating of mis-aligned vertebrae by a doctor of chiropractic is known as a chiropractic **adjustment** and may be accomplished manually (in which case a 'pop' is often heard or felt as the vertebra goes back into position). Gentler chiropractic adjustments may be accomplished with the aid of instruments which 'tap' the vertebra back into position.

Chiropractors are typically thought of as treating only back problems because they concentrate on the spine. This is not so. Because spinal nerves supply energy to the **entire** body, spinal adjustments can affect all parts of the body. The bony structures are adjusted to affect changes in the **nervous** system. The range of disorders that can be treated chiropracticly is very wide, for it is an entire system of health care, albeit a non-medical one.

Most of us have been taught to think of chiropractors as "quacks", as "bone crunchers". It has not been a profession that has enjoyed a great deal of respect. Why? Is it because of lack of training of the chiropractor? Or a lack of efficacy of his techniques? Neither. It has recently come to the attention of the American public that the AMA has conspired to destroy the profession of chiropractic in the U.S. On 8/27/87 Federal Judge Susan Getzendanner found the AMA, along with the American College of Surgeons and the American College of Radiologists guilty of such conspiracy. It was established in this 11 year long trial that the AMA paid a team of over a dozen MDs, attorneys and others to attempt to destroy the chiropractic profession in this country (details available in booklet form through the Motion Palpation Institute, 21541 Surveyor Circle, Huntington Beach, CA 92646, 714-960-6577). This was done with the full knowledge and support of the executive officers of the AMA. AMA agents, dispersed throughout the country, referred to chiropractors as "rabid dogs", "killers", "cultists", "unscientific" and "quacks". These are the actual terms that showed up in AMA documents. On 2/7/90 the U.S. Court of Appeals for the Seventh Circuit upheld the guilt of the AMA, the judge stating that they had acted unlawfully, "violating the antitrust laws by conspiring with its members and other medical professional societies to destroy the profession of chiropractic in the United States." Clearly the AMA has done much to damage the chiropractic profession. Let's look at some of the facts about this health care system and the training of their physicians. The chart below compares the education of a D.C. to that of an M.D.

MEDICAL Class Hours (minimum)	Subject	CHIROPRACTIC Class Hours (minimum)
508	Anatomy	520
326	Physiology	420
401	Pathology	205
325	Chemistry	300
114	Bacteriology	130
324	Diagnosis	420
112	Neurology	320
148	X-ray	217
144	Psychiatry	65
198	Obstetrics & Gynecology	65
156	Orthopedics	225
2,756	TOTAL HOURS	2,887

Other required subjects for the Doctor of Chiropractic: adjusting, manipulation, kinesiology, and other similar basic subjects related to his specialty. Other required subjects for the Doctor of Medicine: pharmacology, immunology, general surgery, and other similar basic subjects related to his specialty.

GRAND TOTAL CLASS HOURS
Including Other
Basic Subjects

4,248   4,485

This data was compiled from a review of the curriculum of 22 medical schools and 11 chiropractic colleges and updated from the National Health Federation Bulletin and other publications' statistics. We can see that the chiropractic student takes **more** hours of anatomy, physiology, bacteriology, diagnosis, neurology, x-ray and orthopedics than does the medical student. This might account for the reason why chiropractors were found (according to testimony given in the trial) to be **twice** as effective as medical doctors in treating musculo-skeletal problems. Many chiropractic colleges require courses in nutrition. While the D.C. can and frequently does utilize and dispense nutritional supplements, he cannot prescribe drugs, nor perform surgery. Such practices are outside of the realm of not only his expertise, but also outside of the philosophy of the profession. At present chiropractors do not generally have hospital privileges.

Today, despite AMA attempts at suppression, chiropractors are licensed in every state and their services covered by insurance. The profession is gaining much earned respect, despite the many obstacles placed before it by the AMA.

OSTEOPATHY

It was an M.D., Andrew Still, who was credited with developing osteopathy in 1874. Osteopathy is based on the theory that sickness is due to sluggishness of the vital body functions. The traditional D.O. therefore practices bodily **manipulation** (much like chiropractic adjustment) to stimulate the circulation of blood and lymph. Dr. Still, though a licensed M.D., insisted that the body needed no drugs. This is the philosophy of traditional osteopathy. However, somewhere along the way, medical practices became intermingled with osteopathic ones. Today osteopaths throughout the country are licensed to practice medicine, including surgery and the prescription of drugs. Certain colleges in the United States are accredited by the American Osteopathic Association to offer the required four year course of training and grant the D.O. degree. These colleges also give complete instruction in conventional medicine. The typical osteopath in practice today has however abandoned clinical use of the manipulation skills which he learned in school and is thus indistinguishable from his medical counterpart. Every now and then we may encounter an "old school" osteopath who still practices manipulation, but he is (sadly) the exception and not the rule.

NATUROPATHY

The term "naturopathy" was coined by John H. Scheel in 1895, but the profession was given its biggest boost by Benedict Lust who came to the U.S. from Germany to introduce the Kneipp water cures. This remarkable man was an M.D., a D.O. and an N.D. He founded the American Naturopathic Society in 1919.

The naturopath is probably the most versatile of the physicians, for he is trained in all forms of **natural** healing (this excludes medicine). We can expect the naturopathic physician to have some knowledge of a variety of treatment and diagnostic modalities which may include bodily adjustments and manipulations, herbology, homeopathy, iridology, acupuncture, nutrition, etc. The D.C. may choose to study and become certified in any of these areas too, but, except for adjustment and manipulation, these subjects are not generally emphasized in his formal training. In theory, the M.D. or D.O. may also become certified in any of these areas. In practice however, he rarely does, for they are not likely to appeal to him (having a different philosophical orientation than medicine) **and**, were he to practice them, he would risk being ostracized by members of his own profession.

At the time that Dr. Lust founded the American Naturopathic Society, naturopathy was a well respected profession that gained in popularity for another decade or so. It was the introduction of the "wonder drugs" (antibiotics) and the widespread acceptance of the germ theory (see chapter 2) as the cause of disease that caused naturopathy to drop in popularity.

Today naturopathy, like chiropractic, is struggling to regain acceptance and is meeting with some success, though it has not made the strides that chiropractic has in the nation as a whole. Only seven states now license naturopathic physicians. Among these are Washington and Oregon, both homes of well respected naturopathic colleges (John Bastyr in Seattle and the National College of Naturopathic Medicine in Portland, founded in 1956). On 6/21/89, John Bastyr College received word of accreditation by the Commission on Colleges of the Northwestern Association of Schools and Colleges. The effective date of NASC accreditation was retroactive to 9/1/88.   JBC has tough admission standards (basically the same as for chiropractic college - AA degree with heavy course work in the sciences) and the curriculum is a demanding one. It includes courses in biochemistry, anatomy, physiology, immunology, microbiology, genetics and nutrition. In fact, John Bastyr offers degrees in nutrition. In Seattle, John Bastyr graduates in naturopathy may practice side by side with medical doctors. This is the type of co-operative interdisciplinary approach to health care that we support and would like to see spread.

If chiropractic, traditional osteopathy and naturopathy, as described above, really are valid alternatives to medicine, why is the public not aware of this? The answer takes us back once again in time:

In the early 1900s the Rockefeller and Carnegie Foundations became quite heavily involved in the practice of giving philanthropic grants to medical schools. Their goal was to create an exclusively male, upper class medical profession rooted in the philosophy of allopathic medicine or drug therapy. In 1909 they sent a man named Abraham Flexner on a tour of all schools involved in health care training. The following year the Flexner Report was issued. After that, the number of medical degree granting institutions in the U.S. dropped from approximately 400 down to 65. By reducing the number of medical physicians, supply went down, demand increased. The medical doctor began building a monopoly over the delivery of health care in the U.S. The Flexner Report dealt a severe blow to all non-medical health care systems, for the Rockefellers and Carnegies, with their legislative clout, were influential in having regulations passed which limited official recognition to the medical approach. The Rockefellers were heavily vested in the pharmaceutical industry.

Apart from the legislative domain, the credibility of medicine is suffering as a consequence of its own failures. Medicine is concerned with the study of disease and suppression of symptoms. We maintain that such suppression is not only not synonymous with a cure, but is actually **dangerous** to the patient. The suppression of disease symptoms through the use of allopathic medicine does not remove the basic cause of the problem, but does, in fact, exacerbate it by driving toxins deeper into the tissues of the body: If we suppress a cold, we may later develop the flu. Suppression of the flu can result in development of pneumonia. Suppression of pneumonia may ultimately lead to bronchitis. Development of asthma can later ensue as a result. Further suppression can manifest as emphysema. This development from acute to chronic disorders has a decided scientific basis as detailed in Homotoxicology by Hans Heinrich Reckweg, M.D. Herein lies the danger of allopathic medicine. Americans are popping 25 million pills per hour and our health is **not** improving. The average hospital patient is given six different drugs. With six different drugs, there is a 100% chance of adverse interaction and the development of serious side effects. We have a word - **iatrogenic** - for those illnesses resulting from the practice of medicine. A study at Boston Hospital showed that 35% of their patients were admitted as a result of development of iatrogenic disorders. Statistics from other sources vary from 15 -

60%. The medical profession stands in violation of its first law: DO NO HARM. The true story printed below in the January, 1974 edition of the magazine Share deals with the possible grave consequences of iatrogenic disease:

THE WISDOM OF ALLOPATHIC MEDICINE

A young man developed a sore throat. He went to his physician who prescribed penicillin for the inflammation. The sore throat promptly disappeared. Three days later, however, he developed itching and hives all over his body. A physician correctly diagnosed a penicillin reaction and prescribed antihistamines. The hives went away.

The antihistamines caused the patient to be drowsy so that he cut his hand while at work. He went to his company's nurse who put some antibacterial salve on the injury. The salve contained penicillin and caused the hives to return.

Recognizing a possible serious anaphylactic reaction for the second time, his physician then prescribed corticosteroids (cortisone). The hives again disappeared.

Unfortunately, the patient developed abdominal pains and noticed blood in his stools. The correct diagnosis was then made of a bleeding peptic ulcer brought on by the cortisone. The patient failed to respond to standard measures to correct the hemorrhage so the next course of action indicated was a partial gastrectomy. The surgery was successful. The stomach pains diminished and the bleeding stopped.

The patient lost so much blood due to hemorrhaging and the stomach surgery that a transfusion was indicated. He was administered two pints of blood and promptly contracted hepatitis as a result of the transfusion.

Being young and vital, he recovered from the hepatitis. However, at the point of insertion of the transfusion needle, a painful red swelling appeared, indicating a probable infection.

Having had a previous bad experience with penicillin, the drug of choice for this infection became tetracycline. The infection promptly subsided.

Disruption of the intestinal bacteria by the tetracycline caused painful abdominal spasms and severe diarrhea. The patient was then administered an antispasmodic type of drug and the diarrhea and spasms subsided.

Unfortunately, this drug was in the belladonna, or muscle-relaxing group of drugs which relaxed the smooth muscles all over the body. From this action on the muscles of the iris of the eyes, it impaired the patients vision. He drove his car into a tree and was instantly killed.

In the above case, at least the diagnoses made of the patient's conditions were correct. This is not always the case. A six year study by Dr. Barkley Sanders for the National Health Institute using 100,000 patients showed that medical doctors were correct in their diagnoses only 20% of the time!

Dr. Hardin B. Jones of the University of California who had been a cancer researcher for over 45 years did a study on patients who didn't listen to their doctor. He found that those receiving conventional treatment lived 4 more years on the average, while those who received no treatment lived an average of 12 more years!

Dissatisfaction with the results of allopathic medicine plus escalating health care costs have caused over 35 million Americans to seek alternatives. 1989 saw a 4% inflation rate, but an 18.9% increase in health care costs. Today an estimated 89% of Americans believe that some fundamental changes must be made in medicine and health care (Wellness Lifestyle, May, 1990). It is highly significant that historically every time and everywhere that doctors have gone on strike the mortality rate has dropped.

On the next page is a reproduction of an admission form used in 1982 in one of our state mental hospitals. Note the array of drugs that may be administered and the host (over 2 dozen) of possible side effects, ranging from increased thirst to death. These side effects are not limited to psychoactive drugs, but may apply to any allopathic medication. Immune suppression is a side effect of three out of four allopathic drugs. It is the responsibility of the M.D. to advise his patients of possible side effects. If your M.D. does not do so, then we suggest it is your responsibility to ascertain them

MEMO   September 22, 1982

SUBJECT: FORM TO BE USED FOR PATIENT CONSENT TO
          MEDICATIONS

I was advised by my physician, Dr. _____, that during my stay here at _____, I might be given one or more
of the following medications.

Thorazine (chlorpromazine)	Serentil (Mesoridazone)
Stelazine (Trifluoperazine)	Lithium Carbonate
Compazine (Prochlorperazine)	Vistaril (Hydroxyzine)
Haldol (Haloperidol)	Pamelor (Nortriptyline)
Librium (chlordiazepoxide)	Artane
Mellaril (Thioridazine)	Cogentin
Navane (Thioridazine)	Bendaryl
Norpramin (Cesipramine)	
Prolixin (oral) (Fluphenazine)	ANTI-CONVULSANTS
Prolixin Decanoate	Tegretol
Presamine (Imipramine)	Clonopin
Sinequan (Doxepin)	Zatontin
Trilafon (Perphenazine)	Dilantin
Valium (Diazepam)	Dilantin c Phenobarbital
Loxitane (Loxapine)	Mysoline
Moban (Molindone HC1)	Tridione
Elavil (Amitriptyline)	

These medications are given to me to calm or quiet my fears, if any, to control unwanted thoughts or voices
if present, and improve my behavior if need be or if I am an epileptic so that I should not have a fit and hurt
myself.

One or more of these medications may have one or more of the following results.
It may:

Hurt my liver
Lower or raise my blood pressure
Make me drowsy
Make me thirsty
Make me have a rash
Make me sensitive to the sun
  or sunburn eadily
Make me have a fever
Make me fat
Make me have blurred vision
Make me turn yellow
  on my face
Make me stagger
Make me have swellings because
  of water in various parts of my body
Make me have pimples or a rash
  on my face
Make me temporarily impotent
Make me react badly to
  alcohol or drugs
Make me have seizures
Make me excited
Make me constipated

Make my face twitch and
  make me chew my tongue
Make my white blood cells low
Make my heart work badly
Make my skin & the whites
  of my eyes yellow
Make my hands shake
Make my body stiff
Make my mouth dry
Make my breasts swell
Make my skin copperish
  or darker
Make my eyes roll up
Make my skin break out in
  reddish patches
Make my walk shuffle
Make the tissues of my
  body sick
Make me die from alcohol or
  street drugs
Make me drool

for yourself by consulting a PDR (<u>Physician's Desk Reference</u>) or a similar publication written for laymen. After reading up on it, if you still choose to take the medicine, fine. If you are wondering what the alternatives are, read on....

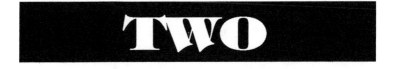

DISEASE CAUSATION

Dr. Harold Reilly in The Edgar Cayce Handbook for Health Through Drugless Therapy speaks about "C.A.R.E.": Circulation, Assimilation, Relaxation and Elimination. If the body is functioning normally in all of these processes, the result is good health. However, if there is impairment in any one of these areas, others will be affected and ill health results, whether or not it manifests in diagnosed disease or even expresses as overt symptoms. Let's look at each component in Dr. Reilly's C.A.R.E. model:

CIRCULATION

Circulation refers to the movement of blood and lymph fluid through the body. The lymphatic system is the life-line of the immune system and is discussed more fully in the next chapter. Circulation of blood provides the oxygen essential for metabolic processes and also removes carbon dioxide, formed as a waste product. Most of us believe that the oxygen we breathe in is exhaled as carbon dioxide. This is not so. Actually, the oxygen unites with hydrogen in the body and is excreted as water through the kidneys. Carbon dioxide is the acid residue produced by normal metabolic processes. We do excrete it, in part, through our exhalations. Acid from foods, however is eliminated through the kidneys, after being neutralized.

The heart is the amazing pump that keeps our blood

circulating. Each day it beats 100,000 times and pumps 4300 gallons of blood. Circulatory problems can result in stroke, heart attack, atherosclerosis (hardening of the arteries) and senility (decreased blood supply to the brain). Since the blood carries oxygen and nutrients to all the cells, impairment in circulation to a given organ or area of the body will result in energy loss at that site. To stimulate circulation, it is helpful to engage regularly in some form of aerobic exercise. Jogging on the rebounder (mini-trampoline) is especially stimulating to lymphatic circulation. Massage, manipulation and the practice of 'dry brushing' the skin also stimulate circulation. A natural bristle, long handled brush is used for dry brushing. The body is brushed vigorously in an upward motion toward the heart from the extremities. This is well to do once or twice daily. A good time is just before showering, for the brushing also removes particles of dead skin. In this manner, the eliminatory function of the skin is assisted.

The flow of blood to the brain is critically important, for interruption of it for just a few minutes can result in a coma; a few more minutes and permanent brain damage is done. So, unimpaired circulation is vital to our health and well being.

<u>ASSIMILATION</u>

Assimilation is the individual's capacity to utilize food. This is a critical function, for even the best of foods will not nourish us if we cannot assimilate, or utilize, the nutrients from it. Assimilation includes absorption, the process by which nutrients are taken up by the intestines and passed into the bloodstream, and the digestive process.

Our ability to assimilate food is largely dependent upon the other three processes in the C.A.R.E. model. Increased circulation will aid in the absorption of nutrients. Thorough elimination is also essential, for incomplete elimination will block nutrient absorption in the intestines and result in lack of nourishment to the rest of the body. Likewise, relaxation permits assimilation, while the stress response inhibits it. When the pH of the body is off balance (see p. 43) assimilation is hampered.

RELAXATION

If we're going to digest our food, it is essential that the body be in a relaxed state at mealtime. Unfortunately, most of us are used to eating on the go and rushing our meals. We learned this at lunch time when we were kids in school. It was often a wait to get through the line in the cafeteria, then a race to consume the food in the allotted half hour. Then we grew up, went to work and got an hour for lunch (some of us), but we're still rushed, for most of us find numerous other activities to cram into our lunch hour. Even if the hour is devoted to eating, it still may be stressful, for many a business deal is consummated at mealtime. Sadly, we are not taught to take our time, sit in silence and savor our food. Meal time is, unfortunately, too often social time and the topics and pace of conversation can be most upsetting to the digestion. Rushed as we are, we do not take the time to thoroughly masticate our food - a few gnashes of the teeth and it's swallowed practically whole, never to be digested, for the process of digestion begins in the mouth, with the secretion of digestive juices. Practitioners of macrobiotics (a Japanese system of living and eating) teach that we should chew each mouthful of food **fifty** times before swallowing it! Try it sometime - even thirty times would be an effort for most of us.

The condition of our mind and emotions at mealtime is extremely important. If we eat when we're tired, angry, excited or under stress, we'll develop indigestion: If we make a habit of it, an ulcer will result.

A relaxed state is facilitated by correct breathing. Deep abdominal breathing relaxes the mind and body and oxygenates the body. Most of us are shallow chest breathers. This habitual aberrant pattern is conducive to a build up of stress in the system. More information on breathing is given in the next chapter.

The body's reactions to stress include (1) rise in blood pressure (2) rise in blood sugar (3) increase in stomach acid (4) constriction of the arteries and (5) shrinkage of the thymus gland. Most of us are familiar with the consequences of the first four effects, but what about the thymus? During the stress response, compounds are released by the adrenal gland that cause this gland to shrink. To understand the significance of this effect, we need to take a closer look at

THE THYMUS GLAND

Our thymus gland is located about an inch beneath the notch where the clavicles come together at the center of the upper chest, just below the neck (where the second rib joins the breastbone). This gland is what is known as sweetbread in calves.

For a long time the standard medical teaching was that the thymus gland has NO FUNCTION. This conclusion was based largely on the fact that autopsies repeatedly showed that the gland was shrunken or atrophied.

In the 1950s it was learned that, not only does the thymus gland have a function, it has a critically important role in the functioning of the immune system. Helper T cells (a form of white blood cell described more fully in the next chapter) mature in the thymus and settle in lymph nodes and cells there. It is the release of the thymus hormone that activates these T cells in the immune response. Without release of this hormone, abnormal cells may not be recognized by the body and diseases such as cancer will spread unchecked, for T cell function (activating the body's defenses) is impaired. So, the health of the thymus gland is imperative to insure the release of its hormone to trigger the immune response. And yet autopsies show shrunken thymus glands. Why? The thymus plays an active role in the growth process, but diminishes in size after puberty when the bulk of growing is done. It has been found that **further shrinkage is due to stress**. Under acute stress, the gland can shrink to half its size within 24 hours. This may happen as a consequence of severe injury or sudden illness. This finding sheds new light on the reason why post mortems consistently revealed shrunken thymus glands. But the effects of stress on the gland were unknown in the first half of this century and when it was discovered that babies who had died of the so-called 'crib death' had **enlarged** thymus glands, it was mistakenly concluded that this thymus enlargement was the **cause** of death. A new disease was thus created: STATUS THYMICOLYMPHATICUS and in the 20s, 30s and 40s children with 'enlarged' thymus glands were treated with irradiation to 'cure' the disorder by shrinking the gland! Whatever effect this may have had upon those children's presenting symptoms, we can be certain that it also gravely damaged their immune systems, making them more susceptible to all manner of infectious disease. Such diseases would be examples of iatrogenic disorders.

The fact that most of us have underactive thymus glands can be demonstrated by a simple muscle test. Put one hand over the thymus area and extend the other (thumb down) to your side. Test the muscle on that arm by having someone apply gentle pressure, pushing the hand downward as you resist. If you cannot resist the pressure when your other hand is over the thymus, but can resist it when the thymus is uncovered, that is an indicator that the energy supply to your thymus gland is reduced. To temporarily increase the energy flow, thump gently on the thymus area with your fists. Make like Tarzan. You should now find that your test muscle is strong when you cover the thymus with the other hand. For more on this subject look into <u>Your Body Doesn't Lie</u> by psychiatrist, Dr. John Diamond.

The power of relaxation to heal is demonstrated through the success of biofeedback. Through this process, which conditions a person to relax, it has been found that control can be gained over autonomic functions, previously thought not to be influenced by conscious thought. People have been successful at learning to control their blood pressure and to diminish and eliminate migraine headaches by learning and applying the relaxation response. Meditation has also been shown to reverse stress reactions.

The power of the mind to heal is becoming increasingly acknowledged. Dr. Carl Simonton has had impressive results in treating cancer patients by teaching them to visualize the healing process. Norman Cousins, in his book, Anatomy of an Illness, highlights the importance of humor and a positive outlook in victory over disease. Faced with an 'incurable' disease, Cousins decided not to let his poor prognosis influence his expectation of recovery. He took responsibility for his health and laughed through the pain - even having Marx Brothers movies brought into his hospital room. This attitude was a significant factor in his recovery, though admittedly nutrition played an important role also.

ELIMINATION

There are four major organs of elimination: intestines, kidneys, skin and lungs. If these eliminating channels coordinate one with the other, then the body drosses are thrown off in a normal way and health is maintained.

We can assist our lungs in the elimination process by practicing deep breathing, utilizing the diaphragm, that large dome-shaped muscle that divides the chest from the abdominal cavity. In diaphragmatic or abdominal breaths, the belly rises as we breathe in, contracts as we exhale - just the opposite of the way that most of us have learned to breathe. As previously mentioned, acid waste is eliminated from the body in the form of carbon dioxide when we exhale. Deep breathing also moves lymphatic fluid, the carrier medium for our immune cells. Many of us are mouth breathers and need to re-learn to inhale through the nostrils, whose tiny hairs filter out airborne particles, preventing them from reaching the lungs. Since the lungs are an organ of elimination designed to assist the body in riding itself of toxins, it is certainly advisable to refrain from adding to their toxic burden by not smoking. There are 47 different toxins in cigarette smoke.

We can assist our kidneys with their elimination function by keeping them flushed through adequate intake of water, a subject covered thoroughly in chapter 6. Adequate intake is generally 1/2 oz. per pound of body weight, although less will be required for the person whose diet consists predominantly of high water content foods (fruits and vegetables and their juices).

We eliminate toxins through the skin when we sweat. Any exercise that causes us to perspire is therefore helpful in this regard. Hydrotherapy, the use of saunas and the practice of massage also stimulate the skin, helping to open the pores and facilitate the elimination process.

The final organ of elimination is the intestines, through which solid wastes are disposed of. Eating a diet high in fiber will facilitate elimination through this channel, for fiber, although it has no nutritional value, acts as sort of a whisk broom in the intestines, sweeping away debris which would otherwise accumulate, causing constipation. A high fiber diet is one that consists chiefly of fruits, vegetables and **whole** grains. Meat has no fiber. Diets consisting primarily of processed, refined foods lack sufficient fiber to keep the colon free of accumulations. As fecal matter and mucous build up in the intestines, the bowel becomes underactive and toxic wastes are then absorbed through the bowel wall and into the blood stream. From there they become deposited in the tissues and this is the beginning of degenerative disease. Accumulations on the bowel wall also become a breeding ground for unhealthy bacteria. The normal balance of intestinal flora (bacteria) is 15-20% putrefactive (harmful, of which e. coli is the dominant strain) and 80-85% beneficial, or of the lactobacillus variety. Antibiotics destroy all bacteria, including the beneficial flora that synthesize B vitamins in the intestines. B vitamin deficiencies may therefore occur after administration of antibiotic therapy if valuable flora are not re-implanted in the intestines. Contrary to popular belief, this cannot be effectively accomplished by eating yogurt, as the dominant strain of lactobacillus in yogurt, bulgaricus, is of animal origin and not viable in the human intestines. Random analysis of stool samples from apparently 'healthy' people have shown a ratio of putrefactive to beneficial bacteria that is exactly the reverse of what it should be: 15-20% beneficial, 80-85% harmful. The proliferation of putrefactive bacteria can cause an overgrowth of the yeast germ, Candida Albicans which can give rise to any manner of symptoms when present in the GI track of men or women. Also, absence of friendly bacteria in the intestines leads to impaired digestion, which in turn can lead to numerous other serious conditions created by the fermentation and putrefaction of undigested food. Undigested food particles in the blood are also a causative factor in the development of allergies.

So - most of us are short on friendly bacteria in the intestines. This shortage is due to many factors - the use of antibiotics, mercury toxicity, the widespread consumption of refined carbohydrates which do not support the growth of valuable intestinal flora, coffee consumption which is destructive to beneficial bacteria.

Because accumulations on the bowel wall create toxic conditions in the body, it is felt advisable, especially for those on the SAD to engage in some form of regular colon cleansing - use of enemas, colonics or colemas (a sort of home colonic unit. See Bernard Jensen's Tissue

<u>Cleansing Through Bowel Management</u> for details on the colema board and the highly effective cleansing program in conjunction with which it is used). Enemas have limited effectiveness because they only cleanse the sigmoid area of the colon (see chart, page 37). Note also that areas of the colon correspond reflexively to areas of the body as a whole. Due to this reflexive relationship, a problem in one area of the body may be caused or perpetuated by an obstruction in that area of the colon that is reflexively related to it. The chart also shows the x-ray outlines of colons of people who thought they were in good health. As you can see, each of these colons is distorted beyond recognition and, although perhaps free of symptoms at the time of the photographs, their owners could hardly be considered 'healthy'. It has been said that health begins and ends in the colon.

If any of the eliminative organs - intestines, kidneys, lungs or skin - are underactive, more wastes are retained in the body. And, as toxins accumulate in the tissues, increasing degrees of cell destruction take place.

Before leaving the subject of elimination, we must say a word about the liver. A major function of this organ is to filter toxins. As long as this function is intact, the bloodstream remains pure. When the liver's ability to filter toxins becomes impaired, toxic substances enter the circulatory system and cause irritation (intestinal inflammation), destruction and eventual death. It has been said that man could live forever if his *liver* kept filtering. We shall look later at ways in which we damage our livers.

Dr. Alexis Carrel of the Rockefeller Institute theorized that the cell could live forever if kept free of its own waste. He designed and implemented a now classic experiment in which the heart tissue of a chicken was immersed in a nutrient solution which was changed daily. He kept the tissue alive for 29 years. At the time of its disposal it was undamaged, youthful and healthy. The results of this experiment went a long way toward proving Dr.Carrel's hypothesis that if the body fluids are kept pure and proper elimination of cellular waste occurs, the cell will live indefinitely. The environment in which the cell lives seems therefore to have a huge amount to do with the health of that cell.

THE PLEOMORPHIC NATURE OF MICRO-ORGANISMS

The medical model of disease causation is based upon the germ theory, the roots of which go back to the middle of the nineteenth century. The principles of this theory were articulated by the famous French scientist, Louis Pasteur, who put forth the notion that specific diseases are caused by specific germs. This concept views germs or micro-organisms as being **monomorphic** in nature, which is to say that they are fixed in form and therefore incapable of changing their identity. A corollary to the germ theory is that specific drugs can destroy specific germs and therefore eliminate the diseases they cause.

In contrast to the germ theory, the natural healing perspective views disease as the result of a process which might be termed **autointoxication**, wherein the body is overwhelmed by its own toxins. This theory is well articulated in the words of Stanley Burroughs from Healing for the Age of Enlightenment:

Disease, old age and death are the result of accumulated poisons and congestions throughout the body. these toxins become crystalized and hardened, settling around the joints, in the muscles and throughout the billions of cells all over the body.

It is presumed by orthodox medicine that we have perfectly healthy bodies until something such as germs and viruses comes along to destroy it, whereas actually the building materials for organs and cells is defective and thus they are inferior or diseased.

Germs in fact are our friends and if given a chance will break up and consume these large amounts of waste matter and assist us in eliminating them from the body. These germs and viruses exist in excess only when we provide a breeding ground in which they can

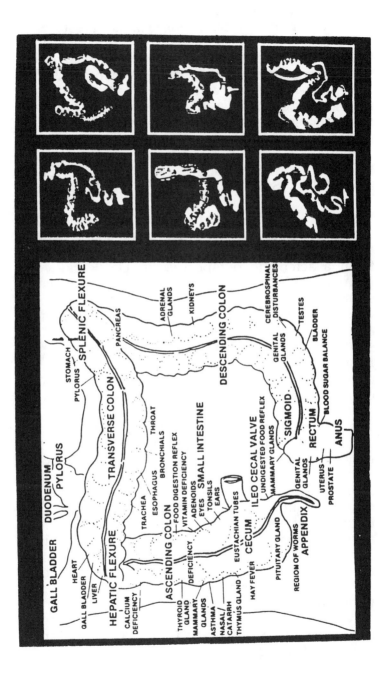

multiply. **Germs and viruses are in the body to help break down waste material and can do no harm to healthy tissue.**

One of Nature's most effective methods of cleansing the body is to start loosening and eliminating these poisons with bacterial action. As this action progresses, we become sick and feverish; large amounts of mucous are eliminated; diarrhea increases the discharge of waste material; and all of our resources go into action to clean out as fast as possible to prevent these poisons from killing us.

INFECTIONS ARE NOT CAUGHT - THEY ARE CREATED BY NATURE TO ASSIST IN BURNING OUR SURPLUS WASTE.

Here we find the notion that symptom formation in the body is goal-oriented and that the goal is healing through cleansing. This concept is explained in detail from a scientific perspective in Dr. Reckeweg's Homotoxicology. The acute symptoms that we so often seek to suppress can be viewed therefore not as illness, but as a "cleansing reaction" or "healing crisis" and should be welcomed as a sign of healing and not suppressed. We should not try to cure a cure! Germs, Burroughs tells us, do not initiate a diseased state, but appear **after** the person has become ill, just as mosquitoes don't cause stagnant water, but are drawn to it.

The natural healing perspective therefore does not deny the existence of germs, but rather asserts that they are basically our friends, serve a constructive purpose in the body and do not create problems for us until and unless a shift or change in the terrain or cellular environment of the host organism causes them to proliferate or multiply - not only to multiply, but also to **change form**. The idea that micro-organisms have the ability to change form is part and parcel of the **pleomorphic doctrine**. In the context of this doctrine a specific germ, let us say an e. coli bacillus, may yesterday have been a bacteria of a different strain and may tomorrow begin to develop into a micro-organism of an entirely different class as a result of changes in the medium (or terrain).

The roots of the pleomorphic doctrine go back in time once again to the middle of the nineteenth century to the work of a Frenchman, Professor Antoine Béchamp, a contemporary of Louis Pasteur. Béchamp held a doctorate in medicine and science, was a master pharmacologist and professor who taught classes in chemistry, toxicology, physics and pharmacology. He was a dedicated man of science who did not seek notoriety, but rather sought to unravel the mysteries of life and, toward that end, spent many hours at his microscope. Pasteur, in contrast (and contrary to what our textbooks tell us) was a rather unremarkable chemist, a second rate scientist with a flare for self-promotion who vigorously sought the limelight and usurped it largely as a consequence of claiming as his own many of the findings of his brilliant contemporary, Antoine Béchamp. These claims are well documented with supporting evidence in Elizabeth Douglas Hume's fascinating book, Béchamp or Pasteur? A Lost Chapter in the History of Biology. Hume emphasizes that, while Pasteur enjoyed popularity with Napoleon and therefore became the "people's scientist", he was not well respected by his scientific colleagues. There is much evidence that Pasteur was in fact a plagiarist and not the brilliant scientist we were taught to believe him to have been. Ironically, his very germ theory resulted from his misinterpretation of Béchamp's early fermentation experiments (see details in Hume's book). While Béchamp theorized the pleomorphic nature of micro-organisms and supported his theory with impressive and convincing experiments, he did not have available to him the technology which would have allowed him to actually witness pleomorphic activity. This technology would be introduced about twenty years after his death by an extraordinary American researcher, Royal Raymond Rife.

Sadly, few have heard of the work of "Roy" Rife. Had his work been acknowledged and applied, disease as we know it today, might have become obsolete. This incredible man made two hugely significant contributions to the field of medicine despite the fact that he was not a doctor. In the late 1920s Rife designed and constructed a light source microscope capable of magnifying, with clarity 17,000X. He later perfected it to magnify to 60,000X. Even more extraordinary than the scope's magnification capacity was the fact that it could be used to examine **living** tissue. Rife stained viruses with **light** to make them visible. Each kind of cell or micro-organism has a specific frequency of interaction with the electro-magnetic spectrum. What Rife did was to "tune into" the natural frequency of the micro-organism, causing a resonance or feedback loop so that the micro-organism effectively illuminated itself. In this way viruses were "stained" with a light frequency just like colors are tuned in on television sets.

Using his Universal microscope, Rife identified the cancer virus in **1932**. No ordinary light source microscope even today would be able to make the cancer virus visible. With his discovery, Rife found that changing the **medium** in which a micro-organism lived would change its form. He thus demonstrated beyond a shadow of a doubt that bacteria are pleomorphic rather than monomorphic in nature. His work highlights the importance of cellular environment or the condition of the terrain or medium. Rife identified four forms of the cancer micro-organism and showed how the virus changes form **depending upon its environment**. He showed that the cancer micro-organism has the ability to change from a bacteria to a virus, depending upon **what it has been fed**. The viral form is one phase in the history of many, if not all, bacteria, he found. The bacterial form of cancer does not produce tumors, but the viral form does. Rife also identified a fungal form of the cancer micro-organism. Any of these forms can be changed back into the viral form with 36 hours and produce tumors. Given Rife's findings, it becomes clear why so many dietary approaches to cancer treatment have been successful - they change the cellular environment so that it is no longer conducive to the development of the viral form of the cancer micro-organism.

Once Rife had observed the cancer micro-organisms with the aid of his microscope he was able to duplicate their frequency. He then went on to develop a frequency instrument that would devitalize them by attuning to that frequency. If all forms of the micro-organism weren't destroyed, the cancer could find another environment in a weakened body and start over again. Terminal cancer patients were being cured in the 30s by being treated for *three minutes every third day* with Roy Rife's frequency instrument. No pain or sensation was experienced - just remission of the disease. It was further demonstrated that any infectious disease could be cured in like manner. Fifty two diseases were being treated successfully with Rife's frequency instrument. Today no library reference to Rife or his microscope exists. His work was effectively buried by the medical establishment to which it posed a threat. The story behind the suppression of his work is told graphically in The Cancer Cure That Worked by Barry Lynes with John Crane, Rife's former lab assistant. Rife's work demonstrates that *it is the frequency of the mass that cures and not the mass itself*, a truth which will be fully developed in this New Age.

As fascinating and important as the frequency instrument is, we would like to focus here on Rife's confirmation of the pleomorphic nature of micro-organisms. This is in sharp contrast to the more widely accepted, traditional view of micro-organisms as monomorphic entitles which says basically that a virus is a virus is a virus and remains so throughout its life. Rife's discovery that a micro-organism can, in effect, change into a entirely different form in as little as 36 hours, depending upon the cellular environment created around it, is highly significant and helps to explain and validate some of the basic premises of the philosophy of disease causation from the natural healing perspective as previously expressed in Stanley Burroughs' quote.

Today there lives and works in Canada an extraordinary French biologist who, despite the fact that he never heard of Béchamp of Rife, unknowingly brought together the work of these two great men through his own research initiated over forty years ago. His story is told in Christopher Bird's wonderful book, The Life and Trials of Gaston Naessens. The Galileo of the Microscope.

Naessens developed on his own a Rife type microscope which allowed him to view the activity of living micro-organisms with complete clarity. Interestingly, this microscope, which he dubbed a somatoscope, is not eligible for patent because it defies the known laws of optics! With the aid of this instrument, Naessens, over the years, has not only viewed pleomorphic activity, but has analyzed this activity and identified its stages of development in healthy and pathological states and has confirmed what Béchamp came to believe over 100 years ago: that the stuff of which germs are made is our own genetic material! Naessens identified a basic life particle which he called a **somatid** and described as a "sub cellular, ultramicroscopic, living and reproducing form that circulates in the blood of all animals and in the sap of plants." This sub cellular life particle is one and the same as the **microzyma** described by Béchamp in his work. Through the crude microscopes of his time Béchamp could not clearly discern the form, but he learned much of its function through his experiments. With the aid of his somatoscope, Naessens could clearly view and study the somatid and even succeeded in culturing it. He considers this life particle to be a precursor to DNA and has found it to be indestructible, as Béchamp had also found. These findings give new dimension to the old adage that "disease is born in and of us", for we have here a model of germs **resulting** from disease rather than **causing** it.

Béchamp, Rife, Naessens and many other researchers over the years have discovered the truth of the pleomorphic doctrine and it is a truth that can no longer be suppressed.

As Royal Rife demonstrated with his frequency instrument, the key to conquering disease lies not in killing germs, but rather in changing the cellular environment from one that is conducive to the proliferation of virulent micro-organisms to one that is not. All forms of natural healing that are successful are successful because they are able to do this.

Whether we change the cellular environment as Rife did through the application of pure frequency (radio waves), or, as many have done, through dietary changes, we devitalize the micro-organism by eliminating the conditions that gave rise to its creation and proliferation. This is vastly different than killing bacteria with chemo-therapeutic agents, a procedure that produces extremely dangerous side effects. Even Pasteur, father of the germ theory, is said to have declared on his death bed: "The microbe is nothing-- the terrain is everything." Unfortunately, medicine sees it differently and it is the system -still- with the monopoly on health care in this country.

No discussion of cellular environment would be complete without reference to:

pH

pH is Potential of Hydrogen ion concentration. It is used to measure the relative acidity or alkalinity of substances by this scale:

0	7	14
acid	neutral	alkaline

As the line indicates, a substance is neutral at 7. Distilled water has a pH of 7. The lower the pH, the more acid the substance.

The pH of our blood is neutral to slightly alkaline. According to the late Prof. Louis C. Vincent, pioneer in bioelectronics, the ideal blood pH lies between 7.0 and 7.2. Any significant deviation from this range is fatal. The organism therefore will go to great lengths to protect the pH of the blood. If it starts to become too acid (as is so often the case with the SAD), then the body buffers it by adding some alkaline minerals - sodium, calcium, potassium, magnesium. If these minerals are not supplied in the diet in a **usable form**, they must be taken from the body's storehouses, its own tissues. The primary alkaline mineral is sodium, which is stored in the liver. When the liver is depleted of sodium, it can no longer neutralize toxic acids and it is at this point that the toxins get into the bloodstream. At this time the endocrine glands take over (primarily the pituitary, thyroid and adrenals) and it becomes their task to direct the toxins to other eliminative organs - the lungs, skin, kidneys. In their efforts to take on this added chore, the glands go first into hyperfunction (overactivity) and then into **hypo**function. In their hyperfunctioning stage, they enlarge and cause disease. In Food is Your Best Medicine, Dr. Bieler (M.D.) points out that the enlarged pituitary can lead to migraines, blindness and epilepsy; hyperthyroidism can give rise to skin and lung diseases, as well as growth disorders and the hyperfunction of the adrenal glands can cause diarrhea and kidney troubles.

When the liver has been depleted of 70% of its sodium (to provide alkaline substance to protect the pH of the blood), then the body stops pulling the mineral from it and goes to the muscles. When the muscles become depleted of sodium, they become flabby. At that point, the body begins to draw on its storehouse of calcium. Tissues, muscles and bones are robbed, giving rise to such degenerative diseases as arthritis, emphysema, osteoporosis and cancer.

We need to clarify that the minerals needed by the body are those of the **organic** form. When we speak of sodium, we do not mean table salt - that is **inorganic** sodium chloride. (A discussion of organic/inorganic minerals can be found in chapter 4.) Much of the food consumed in the SAD is mineral poor and many of the minerals that are supplied are of an inorganic nature and therefore not usable by the body.

When we eat a poor diet and subject the body to other stresses we upset the critical pH balance. Such stress causes a reduction in hydrogen ion concentration in the **tissues** of the body. As the amount of hydrogen decreases, pH (**potential** of hydrogen) increases, creating an alkaline condition in the tissues. Hydrogen ions are then shifted to the **blood**, lowering its pH. It is at this point that the body is forced to draw from its own storehouses of alkaline mineral to protect the critical pH of the blood. Vincent has demonstrated that deviations from the ideal pH in blood, urine and saliva, along with deviations in other parameters (RH2 and R, described in Chapter 6) create different disease patterns.

Many diseases begin when tissue becomes too alkaline, causing a shift in pH in the blood. Alkalinity in an organ or tissue causes harmless micro-organisms to reverse their polarity and become toxic, giving rise to such conditions as cancer. Different body tissues have different pH values. Cells with high metabolic activity normally tend to be acidic due to increased carbon dioxide production, while cells with a lower metabolic rate tend to be more alkaline. A cellular environment that preserves the slight alkalinity of the blood and slight acidity of most of the body tissue appears to be one that is health promoting. The diet that is recommended to maintain or create this desired pH balance is one that is described as approximately 20% acid forming and 80% alkaline forming.

When we say acid or alkaline **forming**, we are referring to the pH created by the foods after they have been digested, not the pH of the foods in their raw state. A food can be acidic in its raw state and yet be alkaline forming. A raw lemon, for example, has a pH of 3, but leaves an ash of 9.

Basically, alkaline forming foods are all vegetables (except legumes) and most fruits. The acid forming foods include sugars, most grains, all meat and fish and most nuts.

Some foods are categorized differently by different authorities. It is generally agreed that millet and buckwheat are the only two grains which are not acid forming, though one authority (Herman Aihara, Acid and Alkaline) lists buckwheat as acid forming. Fresh picked corn is alkaline forming, but generally corn is listed as acid forming, for it becomes so within a short time after being picked. The consensus seems to be that sugars are acid forming, vegetable oils alkaline forming, and nut oils acid forming. Honey is the one sweetener considered to be alkaline forming. There is widespread disagreement on dairy products: We have seen some charts list them as acid forming, some list them as alkaline forming and another as neutral. We believe that the degree of acidity of these products depends upon the extent to which they have been processed and we would therefore list pasteurized dairy products as acid forming and raw ones as alkaline forming.

While nuts are generally acid forming, most authorities seem to agree that Brazil nuts and almonds are exceptions. Another area of disagreement about categorization of acidity/alkalinity is in regard to fruits: While all seem to agree that most fruits are alkaline forming and that cranberries are one exception, plums, prunes and rhubarb are also listed by one source as further exceptions (Dr. Harold Reilly, The Edgar Cayce Handbook for Health Through Drugless Therapy). We cannot reconcile these discrepancies except to state that differences in pH measurements can be the result of use of different measurement techniques and advise that you focus on the areas of agreement and draw your own conclusions re: the exceptions. As regards the plum, while some authorities list it as acid forming, we observe that the Japanese umeboshi plum (used widely in macrobiotics) has an alkalizing effect upon the system. Any fruit when cooked becomes acid forming.

Eggs are generally listed as acid forming. Most grains are acid forming, while seeds (pumpkin, sunflower and sesame) are not. Sprouting both grains and seeds makes them more alkaline. To try to clarify the categorization of foods according to pH, refer to the lists below. The items with the asterisks are those upon which there is not total agreement:

Alkaline Forming
fruits (except cranberries, plums*, prunes*, rhubarb*)
all vegetables except legumes (and most dried peas
    and beans)
Brazil nuts, coconuts and almonds*
millet, buckwheat*
lima beans*
soybeans*
sprouted grains and seeds

Acid Forming
grains (except millet and buckwheat* and corn*)
all poultry, fish, meats and eggs*
sugars and syrups (except honey)
nuts (except Brazils and almonds*)
legumes and beans (except limas* and soybeans*)

There are good wholesome foods in both lists. What we need to aspire toward is selecting more foods (approximately 4/5 of our diet) from the top list. The ideal diet would maintain the gentle alkalinity of the blood and yield a 6.5 saliva value and a 6.8 urine pH, according to Vincent's research. Most degenerative diseases, he established, are the product of high (alkaline) blood and saliva pH and low (acid) urine pH, resulting largely from poor diet.

To get an idea of your body's pH, use special pH paper (which turns a different color for each number - the more alkaline, the darker) to check your urine and saliva first thing in the morning. Check the saliva upon awakening, before rising, and test the first urine of the morning. You will find that the urine pH will change rapidly and vary from day to day, depending upon what you recently ate. During a fast or cleansing diet, it will become temporarily quite acid as acid toxins are dislodged from tissue and carried out of the body. The pH of your saliva will take more time (probably many months) to change, for it more closely reflects what is happening at the cellular level.

It is not desirable to be too acid or too alkaline. Any imbalance stresses the system and ultimately leads to disease conditions. Please remember: When an organ is stressed, it first goes into hyperactivity and then into hypoactivity. Hyper function is associated with overacidity, hypo function with overalkalinity. In the hyper stage, we may well feel energetic, particularly if stimulants such as coffee, alcohol and cigarettes are used), but the net result is fatigue, resulting from decreased electrical energy to the organs. External stimulation is not a viable substitute for internal regulation. And for the body's regulatory functions to remain intact, we must know and follow the laws of the body, particularly as regards the cellular environment we create through the foods we eat and other lifestyle factors.

There are several factors that cause depletion of our alkaline reserve. Among them are:

..... A high protein diet
..... High levels of stress
..... Highly processed foods

To build up our alkaline reserve, we want to:

..... Eat plenty of fruits and vegetables
..... Get fresh air and sunshine

When we exhale, we get rid of 300 times more acid than in any other way, so be sure to exhale completely.

Think of pH as Potential for **Health**. As you succeed in establishing a balanced pH in the body, you will be creating a cellular environment which is not conducive to the proliferation of micro-organisms.

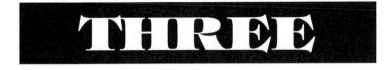

LYMPHOLOGY

The organs of the immune system are generally referred to as **lymphoid** organs. They are concerned with the development, growth and deployment of white blood cells, the most important of which are the lymphocytes. The lymphocytes provide the body's line of defense against antigens. An antigen is any molecule that the body identifies as 'non-self' - virus, bacteria, fungus, parasite, pollen. Even a tissue transplant will be treated by the body as an antigen and rejected unless special measures are taken to bypass the rejection mechanism by suppressing immune function.

The main bases of the immune system are the bone marrow, thymus, lymph nodes, liver and spleen. Auxiliary lymphoid organs are the tonsils, appendix and the Peyer's Patches found in the small intestines. So, the tonsils and appendix, which most of us have been taught have no purpose, and many of us have had removed, are actually part of our immune systems! Their purpose is to assist the body in elimination of catarrh, phlegm and mucous acid. The function of the Peyer's Patches is the collection of toxins.

The lymphatic system itself is the line of supply throughout the immune network. The system is linked up by lymph nodes. These are small structures shaped like beans that are spread throughout the body, concentrated in the groin, abdomen, armpits and neck. The nodes serve as depositories for immune cells and as centers for disposing of the remains of dead microorganisms.

The lifeline for the lymphatic system is a network of vessels similar to, but separate from, blood vessels. These lymphatic vessels contain a clear fluid, lymph, which acts as a carrier for the immune cells. As the illustration on page 54 shows, the lymphatic system looks rather like a tree, with the trunk running down the center front of the body, roots going down into the legs and branches extending into the head and arms. The lymphatic vessels form our 'Tree of Life'.

There are several types of white blood cells or leucocytes, including T cells, B cells and the 'cell eaters' such as macrophages. Special immune cells associated with lymphoid tissue in the body are called lymphocytes. There are two types - T cells and B cells. Think of 'T' as standing for 'thymus'. While all the lymphocytes originate in the bone marrow, helper T cells multiply and mature in the thymus gland. They act as stimulant cells, prompting other immune cells to action when the body's immune competence is compromised by the presence of antigens. These T cells are not themselves fighter cells. They serve more the function of commanding officer or general, mobilizing the troops to fight and calling off the battle (suppressing the immune response) when danger is passed. Other types of T cells do actual hand-to-hand combat, attaching themselves to antigens. T cells called natural killer cells shoot out special proteins which punch holes in antigen walls, thereby killing them.

Think of 'B' as standing for 'bone marrow'. The B cells originate in the bone marrow and mature either there or in immune organs other than the thymus. They are stationary fighter cells and their primary role is the production of antibodies (specific chemical bullets) to fight bacterial invasion. An antibody is a unique kind of blood protein that is synthesized in lymphoid tissue in response to the presence of an antigen and then circulates in the blood plasma. Remember this definition. It is highly pertinent to the discussion of blood proteins that is contained further on in this chapter.

The phagocyte is a special type of cell that patrols the body, hunting down any type of antigen. Consider the phagocytic cells to be the 'Special Forces' or 'Green Berets' of the body's defense system. Macrophages are cells with phagocytic action that hide in the tissues. Monocytes are cells with phagocytic action that hide in the blood. The chart on page 55 shows the action of monocytes on antigens at the site of infection in the body. Note how these phagocytic cells act as killer scavengers, digesting the foreign antigens with Pac-Man like action. After destroying an antigen, the macrophages present a piece of it to the T and B cells who study it and prepare weapons to be used against future invaders.

Most cells of the immune system use chemicals to attack invading organisms. When the invader is encountered, the B cells spawn a multitude of new cells known as plasma cells. Each one of these plasma cells is like a miniature chemical factory. They produce the antibodies which are released into the blood stream. These antibodies will either knock out the antigen or coat its surface to tag it for identification by the phagocyte scavenger cells.

While all of this is going on, the helper T cells oversee the battle, and, if necessary, call in reinforcements. Their function is a critical one, for the immune response would not be evoked without their activity. It is the T cells that are invaded by the AIDS virus. Suppression of the action of these key lymphocytes leaves the body open to all manner of infection, for the B cells will not launch an attack without the command of the T cells.

This cursory overview of immune function prepares us for a look at disease causation at the cellular level and a discussion of

BLOOD PROTEIN RESEARCH

Dr. C. Samuel West helps us to better understand the disease process. His own understanding began in

THE LYMPHATIC SYSTEM

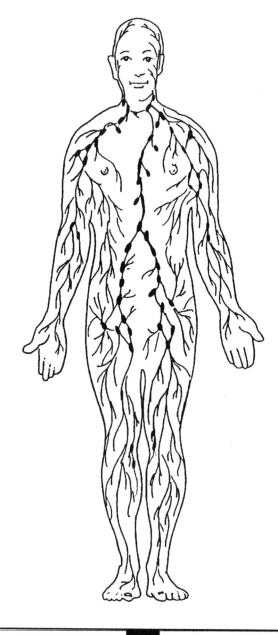

LYMPHATIC ACTIVITY

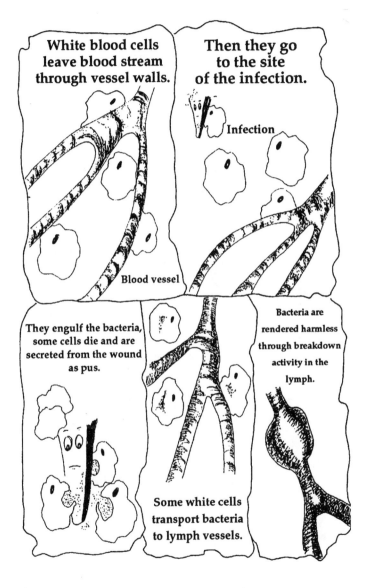

White blood cells leave blood stream through vessel walls.

Then they go to the site of the infection.

Infection

Blood vessel

They engulf the bacteria, some cells die and are secreted from the wound as pus.

Bacteria are rendered harmless through breakdown activity in the lymph.

Some white cells transport bacteria to lymph vessels.

1974 when he learned from the second edition of Arthur C. Guyton's <u>Textbook of Medical Physiology</u> that blood proteins can produce the conditions at the cellular level that can cause death in just a few hours. Over the next six years, Dr. West developed the formula that explains life and death processes at the cellular level. This formula is given and the role of trapped plasma protein expounded upon in his informative book, <u>The Golden Seven Plus One</u>. We attempt in the remaining pages of this chapter to summarize his findings.

Before delving into Dr. West's blood protein research, it is important to understand that everything in the body - all organs, all tissues, hard and soft - is composed of cells. When we fall ill or contract any type of disease or disorder, the cells die or become damaged.

Every cell in the body generates an electrical field. It is an actual electrical generator. We've known for a long time that the thought wave is electrical. It was demonstrated in the 70s in a documentary film that amplified thought waves can influence the activity of matter. In this 'train documentary', electrodes ran from a man's head to an electric train. It was found that the subject could control the movement of the train by thinking about it. His magnified thought waves could stop, start and speed up the electric train. Kirlian photography, developed in the 40s, allows us to view the electrical emanation radiating from all forms of matter. In inanimate objects the radiation or 'aura' is static and, in living beings, it appears as a moving, swirling mass of color and light. Changes in the aura result from changes in our thinking (an electrical phenomenon), among other things. And it has been found that signs of illness show up in the aura before they manifest as symptoms in the body.

Clearly the body is generating electrical current. Our strength and endurance depend upon the energy currents that run through our bodies. In order to keep the electrical generators in the body switched on, two conditions must be met:

(1)   The cells must have sufficient **OXYGEN** and **GLUCOSE**.

Oxygen and glucose are major components in adenosine triphosphate (ATP) production. ATP is the fuel that keeps the generators going. It is the basic energy molecule of the cell.

(2)   The **POTASSIUM** inside the cell must remain high and **SODIUM** low.

Sodium outside the cell wall forces nourishment in. Potassium inside the cell forces waste out. It is the rotation of the minerals in and out of the cell that accounts for its electrical properties. This process of mineral rotation is known as the sodium/potassium pump. **The sodium-potassium pump is the electrical generator in the body.** The sodium-potassium pump is the electrical generator in the body and the ATP turns on the pump. So, without sufficient glucose and oxygen (components of ATP), the electrical generators are not turned on full force and we therefore experience lack of energy. There is a literal short circuit in the body. Now let's look at what is happening on a physical level to produce this condition, which is one of the first symptoms of disease.

Referring to the chart on the following page, we note that section B represents the diseased state at the cellular level. The large white circles in the darkened area are cells. The darkened area itself represents an environment of excess fluid and excess sodium. This condition around the cells will cause them to drown from lack of oxygen (much as a plant dies when we water it excessively) and will upset the delicate sodium/potassium balance in and around the cells. Under these circumstances, the electrical generators cannot be kept going.

To have healthy cells, the body must be able (as shown in section A of the chart) to maintain a negative sub-atmospheric pressure condition or a 'dry state' where

HEALTH   DISEASE

| A | B |

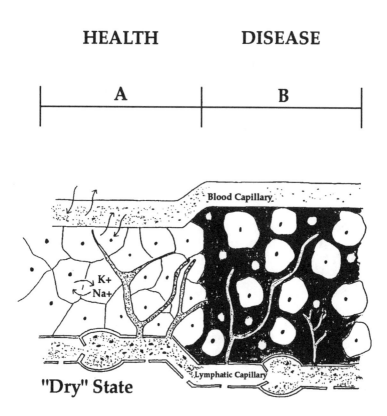

Blood Capillary

K+
Na+

"Dry" State   **Lymphatic Capillary**

Excess Fluid + Excess Sodium = Lack of Oxygen

there is no excess fluid, only enough to fill the crevices around the cells. The sub-atmospheric pressure condition is like a collapsed balloon. In this state the cells remain close together, there is no bloating in the interstitial spaces (between the cells) and the cells remain in close contact with the capillary walls through which they receive oxygen and nutrients carried by the blood. Once the blood deposits these elements, part of it then becomes lymphatic fluid and is recirculated through the lymphatic capillaries.

Referring once again to the chart, the black dots in the blood capillary represent blood proteins - albumins, globulins, fibrinogens - normal constituents of the blood plasma. These blood proteins continually seep through the tiny pores of the blood capillaries into the interstitial spaces. Since there is not enough pressure in these spaces to push the proteins back into the blood stream, they **must be continually removed through the lymphatic system**. Note how the branches of the lymphatic capillary extend like fingers into the interstitial spaces.

Now, if the lymphatic system fails to operate, and the blood proteins get trapped in the interstitial spaces (as is the case in section B of our chart where the small white dots represent the proteins), the result is sickness or death. Death can ensue very rapidly in the case of shock (as Guyton's medical text tells us), where the blood capillaries dilate and dump the plasma proteins into the interstitial spaces all at once throughout the entire system. Since it is a rule that **body fluids follow blood proteins**, water leaves the bloodstream quickly, causing the collapse of the circulatory system. Death can ensue within 24 hours. In the case of degenerative disease, the build up of trapped plasma protein is less rapid and less generalized. The name of the disease will tell us the area of the body in which the blood proteins are trapped in the interstitial spaces.

Once the blood proteins enter the interstitial spaces, if they're not promptly carried off by the lymphatic capillaries, they will cause edema (water-logging) in the spaces between the cells. This is because the proteins carry a negative charge and therefore attract the positive sodium ions from the bloodstream. Remember: *Body fluids follow blood protein.* The main purpose of the blood proteins is to keep water in the bloodstream. However, when they get stuck in the interstitial spaces, the water remains there. And when this is the case, the white blood cells cannot ingest bacteria and impaired immunity results. Remember the definition of 'antibody' given earlier? - "a unique kind of **blood protein** that is synthesized in lymphoid tissue in response to the presence of an antigen and **then circulates in the blood plasma**." Since antibodies are proteins (of the globulin type), they are subject to getting stuck in the interstitial spaces like any other blood protein. When this happens, the body's immune response is suppressed, for it's weapons (antibodies) are effectively unavailable, being 'locked up' in the interstitial spaces.

The condition illustrated in section B of our chart, where we have excess fluid and excess sodium around the cells, upsets the sodium/potassium balance in and around the cells, causes a lack of oxygen and nutrients to the cells and results in loss of energy, inflammation and pain. Excess sodium and lack of oxygen will reduce the electrical energy produced by the cells. Trapped plasma proteins upset the chemical balance of the body and literally cause a short circuit.

When the electrical generators of the body are switched on, we are healthy. **HEALTH IS ENERGY**. It is not merely an absence of symptoms. Many of us consider ourselves to be in good health and yet suffer from fatigue, which is one of the first signs of disease, for it is indicative of reduced electrical potential at the cellular level.

Sodium/potassium balance is critically important in maintaining health, for the sodium/potassium pump is the electrical generator of the body, and when it is switched off, the cells are deprived of oxygen and ATP (fuel for the pump) production is impaired. The late Dr. Max Gerson (whose Mexico clinic has successfully treated many terminal cancer patients through natural means for many years) also recognized the critical role of potassium in the body and taught that loss of potassium from the cells is the beginning of all degenerative disease. Gerson used the potassium in raw foods to correct the deficiency in the body and thus improve cellular respiration, which in turn mobilizes the white cells in their fight against antigens. A special potassium supplement is also used at the Gerson Clinic.

If trapped plasma protein causes disease, then it's logical to assume that we can prevent and possibly reverse the disease process if we know what causes the trapping and how to avoid it. Let's look then at the four basic causes of trapped plasma protein:

POOR NUTRITION

Dr. West tells us that trapped plasma protein is caused by foods that damage cells and make us thirsty. These foods include simple sugars, fats, animal and dairy products and alcohol. These act as poisons in the body. They cause the dilation of the blood capillaries, allowing the blood proteins into the interstitial spaces faster than the lymphatic system can remove them. The ideal diet, Dr. West (and others) tells us, consists primarily of fresh fruits and vegetables and sprouts. Fruits and vegetables are ideal food for five reasons: (1) They are alkaline forming. (2) They are good sources of fiber. (3) They have a high water content. (4) They are an excellent source of glucose (needed for ATP production). (5) They are higher in vitamin and mineral content than any other food.

NEGATIVE MENTAL ATTITUDES

We have already mentioned the fact that shock can cause death within 24 hours by causing the blood capillaries to dilate and the plasma proteins to flood the interstitial spaces, bringing water from the bloodstream with them. On a smaller scale, stress has the same kind of effect upon the body. Negative thoughts act as mental poisons upon the body and cause trapped plasma protein.

PHYSICAL INACTIVITY

Just walking around provides enough stimulation to the lymphatic system to allow for some movement of plasma proteins out of the interstitial spaces. This minimal activity is enough to keep us alive. When we're at rest, the lymph system can drain 1-2 ml. of dead fluid per minute. During activity, it can drain 20 ml. We can therefore see why exercise is important. And there seems to be a special value to aerobic forms of exercise, for "unless we engage in some activity that causes us to breathe deeply, we will have trapped plasma protein, regardless of what else we do" (The Golden Seven Plus One). A gentle bouncing motion, which can be comfortably maintained by doing a 'soft walk' on a rebounder or mini-trampoline is effective in promoting lymphatic circulation. The main function of the lymphatic system is to keep the blood proteins circulating. Exercise assists in this function. The bedridden patient can be benefited by the gentle bouncing motion created by having someone jump up and down on his bed. The wheelchair bound person will reap the beneficial results of someone else jogging on the rebounder if he will place his feet on the jumping surface while the other is doing the exercise. Dr. West makes extensive use of the rebounder in his work and refers to it as a 'lymphasizer'.

SHALLOW BREATHING

The lungs serve as a suction pump for the lymphatics. Deep breathing moves lymphatic fluid very effectively and it floods the cells with oxygen, which enables them to convert glucose into ATP (needed to fuel the electrical generator, the sodium/potassium pump).

According to lymphologist, Dr. Jack Shields, deep breathing drains lymph fluid ten to fifteen times better than any other way.

Most of us do not breathe properly, as was previously discussed. The chest breather never fills his lower lungs, that portion which **should** be supplying 80% of the oxygen to our bodies. Our exhalations are likewise incomplete, which causes us to retain acid waste that otherwise would be expelled in the form of carbon dioxide. Re-birthers tell us that most of us are chronic hypoventilators, taking too little oxygen into our systems. This habit, they say, has its roots in the birth trauma when the doctor held us upside down and smacked our bottoms to shock the system into taking its first breath after the umbilicus had been abruptly severed, moments before. Our first breath, therefore, was associated with trauma. Because of its effect upon lymphatic flow, breath is the major controlling factor in our level of energy and our immune functioning. In a very real sense, oxygen is our most important nutrient. Try breathing in to the count of 5, holding to the count of 20 and exhaling to a 10 count. Your lymph will shoot through the vessels like a geyser. Do this ten times in a row, three times daily. It will nourish and protect the body. If it makes you dizzy, you need it - toxins are being stirred up and removed. Lack of oxygen at the cellular level is a major cause of pain and degenerative disease.

Breath is life. The old Indian, when he was ready to leave his body at the point of death, sat motionless under a tree and took in very shallow breaths to hasten his demise.

We have spoken of trapped plasma protein as a cause of degenerative disease. Before summarizing, we would like to say a few words about injuries: If we accidently smash our thumb with a hammer, what is the first thing that we do, that we instinctively do? We grab the thumb (and say ouch!). But not for long. Soon we let go, reasoning that we should wash it, put ice on it, a band-aid or whatever. And, as we're ministering to the injured finger, what is happening? It is swelling up. Why? Because damaged cells produce poison, histamine. A poison dilates the blood capillaries and lets the blood proteins in faster than the lymphatic vessels can carry them away. A more effective way to handle such an injury would be to continue holding onto the smashed finger. Hold it tightly for up to twenty minutes. Within twenty minutes the poisons have stopped attacking the capillaries. After that, you can let go and do whatever you like and expect to experience little to no pain and swelling.

If poor nutrition, negative mental attitudes, physical inactivity and shallow breathing cause trapped plasma protein, then it stands to reason that exercise, positive thinking, good nutrition and deep breathing will prevent it and help to reverse it. Sustained pressure (as described above) will also help dissipate trapped blood proteins, as will massage and light stroking motions. Electricity has also been found to break up clusters of trapped blood proteins. Clusters tend to form when the energy fields remain reduced in the spaces around the cells and, once they have formed, even the lymphatics have a hard time removing them. In The Golden Seven Plus One Dr. West describes the work of Dr. Joseph Waltz, Director of the Department of Neurological Survey at the St. Barnabas Hospital in New York. Dr. Waltz was able to help patients with cerebral palsy, multiple sclerosis and polio through electrical stimulation of the spinal cord. Also in this book, Dr. West gives us a system of lymphasizing (using the rebounder) designed to maximize lymphatic stimulation, dissipation of trapped plasma protein and pain reduction. He notes that the gentle, bouncing motion on the rebounder creates an electrical field which can be used to magnify thought waves (as was done in the train documentary previously mentioned) and accelerate healing. If the patient will think posi-tive thoughts of healing and direct them at a specific body part, while simultaneously stroking that part and maintaining his 'soft walk' and deep breathing on the rebounder, he can effect positive changes in the targeted body area. See Dr. West's book for details.

It should also be noted that trapped plasma protein can cause obesity. Dr. West states that some people seem to have a 'loose cellular structure' and are therefore very prone to retaining extra water as a result of the blood protein clusters that form readily in their bodies. We can retain up to **21 gallons** of excess fluid in the interstitial spaces - that's a lot of added weight. So, for the sake of your health and your appearance, be aware of the practices that cause trapped plasma protein and consider adopting a more healthful lifestyle.

FOUR

ESSENTIAL NUTRIENTS

VITAMINS

The Concise American Heritage Dictionary defines a vitamin as follows:

Any of relatively complex organic substances occurring naturally in plant and animal tissue and essential in small amounts for metabolic processes.

The Merriam-Webster Dictionary gives us the following definition:

Any of the various organic substances that are essential in tiny amounts to most animals and some plants and are mostly obtained from foods.

Please note the last four words: "mostly obtained from foods". The classical description of a vitamin is a substance which is essential to life and which can be obtained only from outside sources, from food. According to this definition then, a substance may not be regarded as a vitamin if it can be synthesized within the body from the elements obtained from food sources. We have found, however, that certain substances, already classified as vitamins, can be synthesized in the body under optimal conditions. B vitamins are an example. Given the proper balance of beneficial bacteria in the intestines, they can be produced internally. Therefore, our definition of the term 'vitamin' has changed.

Note that each of the dictionary definitions states that vitamins are found in living things and are essential to their existence **in small or tiny amounts**. What is spoken of here is the vitamin in its **natural** form, as it was created by nature, as an integral part of food. The only vitamins that may truly be considered as natural, we maintain, are those which remain unseparated from their food source. Here they exist with other elements with which they work in harmony, synergisticly. In the form of food, nature has provided us with a correct balance of elements, provided the soil from which the food has come is not depleted of nutrients. Soil depletion is a clear and present reality which has given impetus to the trend toward organic gardening. Organic produce is far more nutrient-rich than its non-organic counterpart. (See chart, next page).

Of the less than twenty vitamins discovered so far and believed to be active in human nutrition, we note that most are readily available in tablet or capsule form in mega-potencies. These may well be labeled "all natural". If, as our definitions indicate, vitamins occur naturally in nature in only small or tiny amounts, how, you might wonder, can a high potency vitamin, such as a 500 mg. tablet of vitamin C be "all natural"? The answer is that it cannot be all natural in the sense that it came strictly from a food source, or else it would be larger than a golf ball. Your 500 mg. tablet of vitamin C may have the natural vitamin (from food sources) in it, but it is most assuredly composed primarily of ascorbic acid, the synthetic form of the vitamin. How then can such a product legally be labeled as "all natural"? Easy: Who says "all natural" means the vitamin comes exclusively from food sources? Those who label their products "all natural" are operating within the context of a much broader definition of the word 'natural'. All life on this planet which science recognizes as organic is based on the property of carbon. Carbon occurs in many inorganic compounds as well. It is the primary element upon which life as we know it is based. In this corner of the universe we live

VARIATIONS IN MINERAL CONTENT IN VEGETABLES

Firman E. Baer Report, Rutgers University*

	PERCENTAGE OF DRY WEIGHT		MILLEQUIVALENTS PER 100 GRAMS DRY WEIGHT				TRACE ELEMENTS PARTS PER MILLION DRY MATTER				
	Total Ash or Mineral Matter	Phosphorus	Calcium	Magnesium	Potassium	Sodium	Boron	Manganese	Iron	Copper	Cobalt
SNAP BEAN											
Organic	10.45	0.36	40.5	60.0	99.7	8.6	73	60	227	69.0	0.26
Inorganic	4.04	0.22	15.5	14.8	29.1	0.0	10	2	10	3.0	0.00
CABBAGE											
Organic	10.38	0.38	60.0	43.6	148.3	20.4	42	13	94	48.0	0.15
Inorganic	6.12	0.18	17.5	13.6	33.7	0.8	7	2	20	0.4	0.00
LETTUCE											
Organic	24.48	0.43	71.0	49.3	176.5	12.2	37	169	516	60.0	0.19
Inorganic	7.01	0.22	16.0	13.1	53.0	0.0	6	1	9	3.0	0.00
TOMATOES											
Organic	14.20	0.35	23.0	59.2	148.3	6.5	36	68	1938	53.0	0.63
Inorganic	6.07	0.16	4.5	4.5	58.8	0.0	3	1	1	0.0	0.00
SPINACH											
Organic	28.56	0.52	96.0	203.9	237.0	69.5	88	117	1584	32.0	0.25
Inorganic	12.38	0.27	47.5	46.9	84.6	0.8	12	1	19	0.3	0.20

*This report is not recent. It is over 40 years old.

in carbon bodies. That which is 'natural' to us is that which is carbon based. In a very broad sense, synthetic vitamins can be considered "all natural" since they have a coal tar base. The FDA allows anything containing only 5% natural ingredients to be called 100% natural.

In the natural vs. synthetic controversy, the pro-synthetic argument is made that both forms of the vitamin are chemically identical. The pro-natural side says yes, **but** the vitamin, in its natural form, is found in a food substance that contains other elements which are essential to the proper activity of the vitamin. To extract the single vitamin and greatly increase its potency by the addition of its synthetic counterpart also would disrupt nature's balance of elements, tipping the scales in favor of the vitamin, with little or none of the synergistic elements being provided. We may well be correcting one deficiency, while simultaneously creating others. Science is forever looking for the 'active ingredient' in the products of nature. Could it be that the curative power of the whole food lies instead in its very wholeness? We think so. And, we would have you recall the words 'small' and 'tiny' used in the definitions quoted at the beginning of this chapter. We live in a society that promotes the idea that 'more is better' which is not necessarily so, as the system of homeopathic medicine proves. Whole foods have both a *synergistic* and *molecular* structure. When single nutrients such as vitamins are extracted from food, the *synergistic* structure is destroyed. The isolated vitamin becomes a single chemical, lacking in life force and difficult for the body to utilize. Although chemically identical, it has been established that the atoms in a synthetic product rotate differently than the atoms of a natural one and that the natural product has a more dynamic energy pattern.

We would not want to give the impression that we are unreservedly opposed to the use of vitamin tablets or capsules. It is our belief that where there is a demonstrated deficiency of a specific vitamin, it may be useful to supply it in its concentrated form until the natural balance of elements can be restored through dietary control. We would add, however, that supplements can serve as a dross in a toxic-laden body. Cleansing is a pre-requisite to building or re-building, for without the ability to assimilate nutrients, it is superfluous to supply them in abundance.

If we do choose to take vitamin supplements, we feel that it is essential to have a reliable means of determining what our deficiencies are and what amounts are needed. There is no generally accepted way of doing this. The guideline given to us by the government for the amount needed of each of the vitamins is known as the Recommended Daily Allowance (RDA). The RDA was established by the Food and Nutrition Board of the National Research Council. It specifies a given amount of milligrams, micrograms or units needed for children and adults for each of the vitamins and many of the minerals. The RDA is often criticized for not taking 'biochemical individuality' into account. This is a term coined by Dr. Roger Williams, which reflects the notion that each of us is a unique individual with a unique body chemistry and therefore with individual and unique nutrient requirements. The RDA of one vitamin might be more than sufficient for one person, while quite inadequate for another. Williams suggests that some of us may have inherited a higher than average need for particular nutrients.

Vitamins function with chemicals called enzymes (discussed in the next chapter). Protein molecules, together with substances known as coenzymes make up enzymes. The coenzyme portion is frequently a vitamin. Vitamins and minerals act as catalysts for numerous biological reactions. Vitamins and minerals exist together and work together - vitamin C, for example, increases absorption of iron and the B complex of vitamins is absorbed only when combined with phosphorus.

There are two categories of vitamins - water soluble

and fat soluble. The water solubles are not stored in the body. The tissues absorb what they can use and the rest, we are told, is harmlessly excreted in the urine. However, if the body is overloaded with excessive amounts of a water soluble vitamin, a burden is put on the organs of elimination to excrete the excess. Vitamin C and the B complex are water soluble. Because they are not stored in the body, it is necessary to continuously replenish the supply. Frequent doses are preferable to single ones.

The fat soluble vitamins include A, D, E, K. They are measured in units or international units (IUs), while the water solubles are measured in milligrams (mgs.) or micrograms (mcgs.). The fat soluble vitamins are stored in the body and for that reason, toxic overload is possible, but only probable if one is taking massive doses over a prolonged period of time. The fat soluble vitamins may be administered in single doses daily, since any excess is stored, rather than eliminated.

It is not within the scope of this book to cover each of the individual vitamins, although we do discuss the water solubles in chapter 8. We recommend that the reader become familiar with the food sources of each of the vitamins, as well as deficiency symptoms of each. There are several good reference books which supply this information, among which is the Nutrition Almanac. As you familiarize yourselves with this information, it is well to bear in mind that fruits and vegetables are the major source of vitamins and minerals, fruits being a particularly rich source of vitamins.

MINERALS

Minerals are nutrients that exist in the body and in food. They are found in both organic and inorganic combinations. As with vitamins, it has traditionally been thought that all minerals must be taken in from outside sources, that the body does not manufacture its own. While vitamins can be synthesized by living matter and minerals cannot, the findings of French scientists indicate that biological organisms display the ability to transmute one mineral into another within the cell. Silica, for example, can be transmuted or converted into calcium (see Louis Kervran's <u>Biological Transmutations</u> for more information on this subject). Also, the late Dr. Carry Reams, biophysicist who developed the Biological Theory of Ionization (BTI) maintained that, given certain minerals (calcium, phosphorus, potassium and iron), the body could obtain the other essential ones from the air. So, once again, traditional concepts are being challenged in the face of new ideas and discoveries.

Vitamins, previously discussed, are required for every biochemical activity of the body. They cannot function, however, unless minerals are present. Some minerals are part of vitamins. For example, vitamin B1 contains sulphur, B12 contains cobalt. Although only 4-5% of the body weight is mineral matter, these nutrients are critically important. All of our tissues and fluids contain some mineral. Minerals help maintain water and pH balance. They assist in antibody production. Hormonal secretion of glands is dependent upon mineral stimulation. In fact, all bodily processes depend upon the action of minerals.

There are 84 known minerals, 17 of which are considered to be essential in human nutrition. If there is a shortage of just one of these, the balance of activity in the entire system can be thrown off. A deficiency of a single mineral can negatively impact the entire chain of life, rendering other nutrients ineffective and useless.

Macrominerals are measured in milligrams. They are needed in substantial amounts by the body and include calcium, magnesium, phosphorus, sodium, chlorine, sulphur and potassium. The remaining minerals, needed in small, sometimes minute amounts by the body, are known as trace minerals and they are measured in micrograms. They include iodine, selenium, chromium, copper, etc. There is another class of minerals, known as 'heavy metals' which are toxic to the body. These are discussed separately in chapter 12.

To increase the electrical potential or life force within each cell of the body, one must first have a balance of **USABLE** minerals. This brings us to a discussion of organic and inorganic minerals. Inorganic minerals come from the earth, from soil and rock. They include the carbonates, sulfates, phosphates and oxides, all of which are poorly utilized by the body. They are not absorbed well. If they were, we could eat dirt as a direct source of our minerals! The fact is, however, that we cannot be nourished by dirt, nor can we be nourished by stones or shells which are ground up, no matter how fine. Just because we can swallow them, it doesn't mean that we can utilize or assimilate them. Plants have the capacity to fully utilize inorganic minerals, however, and once they have done so, they have converted them into an **organic** form which is usable by the human body. A mineral is organic when it has become incorporated into living tissue. We can fully utilize the organic minerals found in plants in their raw state. Minerals are rendered inorganic however once heat is applied in the cooking process.

A mineral in its inorganic state has to be **bound to an organic molecule** before it can pass through the intestinal wall into the bloodstream and on to the cells. This binding of an inorganic mineral to an organic molecule is known as *chelation.* When a mineral is chelated, it is altered so that it can be more readily absorbed by the body. When an inorganic mineral is chelated, it is completely surrounded by organic material, held in the 'claws', so to speak, of the organic material (the word chelate means 'claw'). Man has developed the ability to chelate mineral supplements (process detailed in chapter 7) so that they will be better assimilated. The chelated mineral will target the cell, and a certain percentage of that mineral will be fully utilized. When inorganic minerals are consumed, the body cannot assimilate them and may form deposits of the unused mineral material which leads to development of functional disorders (see chapter 6). Now, the human body has the capacity to chelate a small amount of inorganic minerals on its own IF enough hydrochloric acid (HCl) is present. HCl is the acid that *ionizes* a mineral. Ionization is the charging of an electrically neutral substance, giving it a positive or a negative charge. Organic minerals don't need to be ionized. However, inorganic ones must first be separated from their inorganic bonds so that they can be chelated with an amino acid. Amino acids are the most commonly used chelating agents. They are the organic matter best suited for the chelation process.

According to Senate document #264, **99%** of Americans are mineral deficient. Let's look at some of the causes of this deficiency:

(1)   **Insufficient HCl**. Most of us have inadequate amounts of HCl in our stomachs due to excessive intake of protein. Most protein foods are highly acid forming and demand lavish secretions of HCl from the stomach. Over a period of time, the production diminishes, as the organ goes into hypo function. HCl must be present for the body to do its own chelating of inorganic minerals. In its absence, those minerals consumed will not be utilized, producing a deficiency.

(2)   **High Fat Intake**. The excessive amount of fat consumed in the SAD causes ionized minerals to bind themselves to fats instead of amino acids, making them unavailable for absorption into the intestines.

(3)   **Overconsumption of Sugar and Meats**. Both sugar and meat are acid forming. As previously pointed out, when the pH of the blood begins to become too acid, it must be balanced with alkaline minerals. If these are not provided from an external source, the body's storehouses are robbed, resulting in mineral depletion and deficiency.

(4)   **Lack of Enzymes**. The SAD is enzyme poor for

reasons cited in the next chapter. Lack of enzymes in our diet makes it difficult for the body to extract minerals from food.

(5) **Mineral Deficient Soils**. Dr. Reams put forth the theory that all disease results from mineral deficiency. He also demonstrated how depleted our soils have become due to faulty agricultural practices and offered means of accurately measuring mineral content of soil and assessing the degree of mineralization of foods coming from it. Re-mineralization of our soils is essential to the production of a nourishing food supply. The average fruit or vegetable of today does not have the high mineral content of its turn-of-the-century counterpart. More of the same food item would have to be consumed today to provide a mineral content equivalent to the same food of the early 1900s.

Even in our efforts to cleanse and re-build the body, mineral deficiencies can occur, for minerals are rapidly depleted during detoxification and tissue rebuilding. Basically, fruits are the cleansers of the body (citrus being the most aggressive in this activity) and vegetables are the builders. Vegetables are our major source of minerals. Fresh vegetables and their juices supply the body with an abundance of organic minerals with which it can rebuild tissue. Canned and frozen vegetables and bottled juices do not have this capacity, for they have been processed with heat, which converts the organic minerals into inorganic, or dead ones. Life cannot be built from death.

Dr. Paul Eck has demonstrated that not only mineral deficiencies, but aberrant mineral ratios can adversely affect our health. The metabolic rate of an individual can be ascertained by analyzing mineral ratios measured through hair analysis (see chapter 12) and can be corrected through mineral balancing. According to Dr. Eck, restoration of health is dependent upon restoration of optimal mineral levels and ratios. Certain mineral patterns on a hair analysis reflect poor assimilation and slow metabolism, leading to a build up of mineral deposits in the body. Random supplementation can do more harm than good according to Eck because this can contribute to further distortion of mineral patterns. "The way people go about choosing supplements, they could do almost as good using a roulette wheel" (Dr. Eck, The Healthview Newsletter, issue #27-29).

<u>PROTEIN</u>

Adelle Davis, who did so much to awaken public awareness on the subject of nutrition in the 60s, was an advocate of the high protein diet. So were the leading authorities in the field at that time. And as public awareness tends to lag behind current research, so too does the knowledge of today's man-in-the-street. Adelle Davis died in her 60s. She died of bone cancer.

There was a great deal of truth in most of what Davis taught, but her perspective on protein - the old 'more is better' philosophy again - proved to be a fatal error. And sadly, even today, with volumes of research supporting the detrimental effects of overconsumption of protein, the average person still seems to think that he must guard against a protein deficiency and eat plenty of meat to build strength. Ironically, the truth is that protein poisoning is a major cause of degenerative disease today.

The foods highest in protein are meat, dairy products, nuts and legumes. This means they have a very high percentage of protein composition. Fruits and vegetables, while not noted as having a large percentage of protein, do contain amounts that are adequate to meet the body's needs in most cases. And, their protein is of high quality, so that the body may fully utilize it. At one time, it was taught that vegetable proteins were inadequate because they were incomplete - i.e., did not contain all of the 23 known amino acids. We were told that if we were going to 'risk' being vegetarian, we had better combine our vegetables with other foods that provided those amino acids missing from the vegetables. We now know that this is inaccurate, that the body has a circulating pool of amino acids from which it can draw at any time as needed. The body adjusts to whatever amount of protein is available to it. Our cells store protein (which is released from the cells of defective tissue during a fast to be re-built into healthy cells).

Protein is *useless and toxic* to the body unless it is broken down into its constituent amino acids. It is these amino acids which build tissue and strengthen cells. The intake of large amounts of protein is by no means assurance that the body will be able to break it down into amino acids. In fact, overconsumption of protein causes many undesirable conditions including kidney damage, osteoporosis, arthritis, atherosclerosis, immune deficiency and, in the words of William J. Mayo (founder of the Mayo Clinic), "overconsumption of protein has been linked to breast, liver and bladder cancer and leukemia." Let's take a look at the link between high protein intake and disease formation:

As you're aware from information previously presented, most of our high protein foods are acid forming in the system. When the body becomes too acid, toxic build up occurs, for toxins are of an acid nature. When there is an acid build up, the system retains water to neutralize it, as in Dr. West's 'trapped plasma protein' model. Meat and dairy products, you will recall, are among the foods that produce trapping of blood proteins, the beginning of disease at the cellular level. These are, of course, foods that are high in protein.

Excess consumption of protein also causes overstimulation of the pancreas, resulting in reduced enzyme activity. Since enzymes are needed to break foods down into their constituent parts for digestion, the result is poor digestion of proteins into amino acids. Protein then becomes a poison to the body which has difficulty producing adequate enzymes, hormones, antibodies and new tissue. Excessive demands are therefore made on vitamins and minerals (especially B6, zinc and magnesium), leading to nutrient deficiencies. The net result is impaired immunity which can lead to all manner of infectious disease.

Meat contains uric acid - that is acid from the urine of the animal which permeates its system when it is slaughtered. It's the urine which gives flavor to the meat. When uric acid builds up in the system, the kidneys become enlarged trying to process the excess nitrogen. Humans do not have the enzyme, uricase, needed to break down uric acid. Our bodies simply cannot handle it. A build up of uric acid causes such conditions as gout and arthritis.

The more meat we eat, the less acid the stomach becomes. Sufficient stomach acid is necessary for proper digestion of protein. Carnivores have stomach acid which is twenty times stronger than that of humans.

Meat is a food that contains no fiber and is low in water content. Therefore, it clogs the colon, adversely affecting elimination (causes constipation) and assimilation.

Overconsumption of meat and other high protein foods also causes depletion of our alkaline reserves, as has been previously demonstrated. The less alkaline reserve we have, the less protein we can tolerate. Most of us know that calcium deficiency is the basic cause of osteoporosis. And we're taught that we need to take in more dairy products to remedy this deficiency. That is a totally erroneous teaching which will be explored in more detail in chapter 7. A major reason that we become calcium deficient is that we take in too much protein (including dairy products) which causes an over-acid condition, necessitating the robbing of the body's storehouses (bones and other tissue) to buffer the acidity with an alkaline mineral, calcium.

Protein requirements are not the same for all of us.

They vary according to the nutritional status, body size and activity of the individual. The National Research Council recommends the daily consumption of 0.42 grams of protein per pound of body weight. That would be an intake of 75 grams for an individual weighing 150 lbs. This is basically the same recommendation that Adelle Davis was giving in the 60s: consumption of 1/2 gram of protein per pound of body weight. An intake of 25-50 grams of protein per day is, however, adequate for most people. (A 4 oz. serving of meat has about 20 grams). Beyond that amount, we are subject to development of the conditions described above, as well as **declining** strength and endurance. Dr. Irving Fisher of Yale University conducted tests in 1906 and 1907 which demonstrated that vegetarians have almost *twice* the endurance of meat eaters. Fisher's findings were confirmed by Dr. J.H. Kellogg of Battle Creek Sanitarium in later tests. The average American on the SAD, however, takes in between 90 and 100 grams of protein daily. This is unequivocally excessive. It has been found that consumption of more than 6 oz. of animal protein cuts **oxygen intake by 60%** ("Ten Keys to Health", Anthony Robbin's 'Fear Into Power' and 'Nutrition' seminar, 1985). Oxygen, you will recall, is essential to ATP production and therefore to creation of energy at the cellular level. Also, cancer cells thrive where oxygen is undersupplied.

Another way of estimating the body's protein needs is to take a look at how much protein is supplied during infancy, a time of maximal growth, when the body is being nourished by mother's milk. If high amounts of protein were needed to promote growth and strength, we would expect to find mother's milk to be quite high in protein. It is not. It is 2.38% protein, decreasing to 1.2 - 1.6% protein within 6 months of the baby's birth!

The stereotyped image of the caveman is one of a brutish-looking creature carrying a club and gnawing on the carcass of a freshly killed animal. An article appearing in the 5/15/79 edition of the <u>New York</u>

<u>Times</u> tells us this image is incorrect. Dr. Alan Walker, John Hopkins University anthropologist, found that our ancestors were not carnivores, but rather subsisted chiefly on fruit. He drew this conclusion by studying the striations on the remains of their teeth. Fruit then is what we're biologically adapted to eat, what we ate for millions of years. Anatomically, we do not resemble the carnivore. The chart on page 82 compares the anatomy of humans with that of carnivores, herbivores and fruitarians. It is easy to see whom we most resemble. One of the most striking points of comparison is between the intestinal tracts of carnivores and humans. Their intestinal tracts are approximately three times the length of their bodies. Ours are approximately ten times the length of our bodies. They have a short, fast gut. We do not. Meat is very hard for us to digest, and takes longer (5 - 6 hours) than any other food. It stays in the intestinal tract long enough for it to putrify or rot. Putrified food creates acid toxins that the body must buffer with alkaline mineral taken from its storehouses if such mineral is not supplied in the diet.

We tend to equate meat-eating with strength, and yet the strongest animals in the world are vegetarians. Consider elephants and horses. And the gorilla that subsists chiefly on vegetatian (supplemented by small insects). All carnivores find it necessary to sleep 16-18 hours daily due to excessive toxins. They have a very short life span.

In addition to the detrimental effects of meat previously mentioned, we might add that it contains staggering amounts of putrefactive bacteria. Putrefactive bacteria are colon germs and they are liberated from the intestines at the time the animal is slaughtered, permeating the entire carcass. Meat, we all know, is high in saturated fat (see chapter 5) which can lead to many health problems. Overconsumption of it can also lead to a calcium/phosphorous imbalance, with too much phosphorous leading to calcium deficiency. Also, ammonia, a by-product of meat metabolism, is highly

COMPARISON CHART

MEAT EATER	LEAF/GRASS EATER	FRUIT EATER	HUMAN BEINGS
lion, dog, hyena, wolf, cat	cow, camel, elephant, sheep, ox, llama, deer, rhinoceros	ape	man
has claws	no claws	fingers adapted to pick fruit	fingers adapted to pick fruit
sharp, pointed front teeth to tear flesh	no sharp, pointed front teeth	no sharp, pointed front teeth	no sharp, pointed front teeth
no flat back molar teeth to grind food	flat back molar teeth to grind food	flat back molar teeth to grind food	flat back molar teeth to grind food
acid saliva & urine. No ptyalin to predigest carbohydrates	ptyalin present to pre-digest carbohydrates	ptyalin present to pre-digest carbohydrates	ptyalin present to pre-digest carbohydrates
small salivary glands	well-developed salivary glands needed to pre-digest grains and fruits	well-developed salivary glands needed to pre-digest fruits and nuts	well-developed salivary glands needed to pre-digest fruits and nuts
rough tongue	smooth tongue	smooth tongue	smooth tongue
strong HC1 in stomach to digest meat, bone, etc.	stomach acid 20 times less strong than meat eaters	stomach acid 20 times less strong than meat eaters	stomach acid 20 times less strong than meat eaters
short, fast gut; intestinal tract 3 times length of body	intestinal tract 10 times body length	intestinal tract 12 times body length	intestinal tract 12 times body length
simple, round stomach	three compartment stomach	stomach with duodenum (as 2nd stomach)	stomach with duodenum (as 2nd stomach)

toxic and carcinogenic. Add to all of this the risk of developing trichinosis or salmonella from consuming undercooked or spoiled meat and it becomes considerably less appetizing! In summation then, meat-eating leaves a toxic residue of metabolic wastes in the tissues, causing autotoxemia (self-poisoning), overacidity and nutritional deficiency.

The average American eats 150 lbs. of pork, beef and other red meat per year. We would be well advised to reduce our consumption. Meat is a highly stimulatory food, however, and to give it up all at once and totally, could be devastating for the person used to taking in large amounts. To do so would likely produce an overwhelming cleansing reaction (healing crisis) which would be far from being in the best interests of the individual. We recommend, therefore, that the withdrawal be made slowly, over a period of time, to give the body a chance to adapt. We advise that meats be avoided in this order:

.....ground meat (it spoils faster both inside and outside of the body than do other meats)
.....smoked and charcoal meats (use wood chips and don't burn)
.....bacon and other high fat meats
.....whole pork
.....whole beef
.....poultry (remove the skins before cooking)
.....fish (those with fins are best - avoid the scavenger fish: shellfish, scallops, lobster, shrimp)

Whenever possible, it is recommended that organic meats be purchased. These are from animals which were well nourished and not shot up with antibiotics, steroids, etc. Whatever meats you are still including in your diet, it is of utmost importance to consume them in moderation. We know of one patient who, having given up red meat to improve his health, substituted chicken and ate it for every meal. Within a short period of time, he began to lactate! - the estrogen injected into the animal had entered his bloodstream. With the contamination of our planet's oceans, fish is no longer a safe bet either. Avoid entirely those fish, such as tuna, known to be contaminated with mercury. Consider also the way in which your meat is prepared. Do you like it rare, medium or well done? Your response to this question is a good indicator of your level of health, for the more well done the meat, the more acid forming it becomes.

In closing this chapter, we would like to observe that the central element of protein is carbon. And carbon is made up of **six** electrons, **six** protons, and **six** neutrons...**666**...(the 'mark of the beast', Rev. 13:38).

FIVE

MORE ESSENTIAL NUTRIENTS

ENZYMES

In chapter 4 we covered vitamins, minerals and protein - three of six traditionally recognized essential nutrients. The other three are fats, carbohydrates and water. So, what are enzymes doing in a chapter on essential nutrients? They may be considered as a subcategory of proteins, for they are protein-like substances and are considered by some experts to *be* protein. However they are categorized, they are certainly essential nutrients, for it is their job to structure the previously discussed proteins, vitamins and minerals into blood, organs and tissue. Enzymes are found in plant and animal cells and act as organic catalysts in numerous chemical reactions. Their role as catalyst is well known. However, Dr. Edward Howell, biochemist and pioneer in the study of enzymes, who has studied them since 1932, maintains that they are more than mere catalysts, for catalysts are inert substances. Enzymes are not inert, for they radiate life energy.

Although so small as to be invisible, even with the most powerful microscopes, enzymes are the basis of all metabolic activity. They facilitate more than 150,000 biochemical reactions and empower every cell in every tissue, gland and organ of the body to function. Enzymes are responsible for the oxidation process in the body. They are a major factor in such processes as growth, metabolism, digestion and cellular reproduction. More and more enzymes are being identified.

So far, scientists have identified about 2000. Enzymes help extract chelated minerals from food and aid in breaking proteins down into amino acids. Without them we could not breathe, see, digest food or move around. It is enzyme activity that causes food to ripen and spoil and beer to ferment.

There are three classes of enzymes: metabolic, digestive and food enzymes. It is the metabolic enzymes that run our bodies. They do the structuring of protein, fat and carbohydrates and are responsible for the repair of tissue damage in the healing process. Our health depends on an adequate supply of metabolic enzymes. Every organ has its own specific metabolic enzymes to perform specialized functions.

The digestive enzymes digest our food. There are three main classes of digestive enzymes: <u>proteases</u> (that digest protein), <u>amylases</u> (that digest carbohydrate) and <u>lipases</u> (that digest fat). Food enzymes, found in raw foods, start the digestive process in the body and help take the load off of the digestive enzymes. In 1943 the Physiological Laboratory of Northwestern University did experiments on rats which resulted in the development of the 'Law of Adaptive Secretion of Digestive Enzymes'. This law states that the organism will manufacture enzymes *only in the amount needed for any job.* If raw foods are consumed, they will be partially digested by their own food enzymes and the body therefore will make less concentrated digestive enzymes. This law has been confirmed repeatedly through numerous studies in university laboratories. As the law implies, the body values its enzymes. Dr. Howell maintains that all living organisms have a **fixed enzyme potential** and that this enzyme potential diminishes with time. When it is exhausted, life ceases. Our enzyme potential is like a bank account. We can choose to withdraw from it frequently or to save and conserve our precious life sustaining enzymes. Most of us unknowingly are reckless spenders of enzymes. The ingestion of only cooked food demands lavish enzyme secretions from the digestive organs. When we eat cooked food exclusively, we are not taking in any food enzymes with which to digest it and so the body is forced to produce large amounts of digestive enzymes, thus enlarging digestive organs, especially the pancreas, according to Dr. Howell.

The digestive process requires more energy than any other bodily process. Due to faulty eating habits, such as poor food combining and overconsumption of proteins, most of us have food in our stomachs all the time. Our energy is therefore tied up in the digestive process continually, so that there is very little left for other activity. With so much digestive activity going on constantly and excessive amounts of digestive enzymes being made continually, the body becomes unable to produce an adequate quantity of metabolic enzymes needed for fighting disease and repairing organs. This depletion of metabolic enzymes, due to the body's excessive demand for digestive enzymes, is cited by Dr. Howell as a probable cause of many chronic degenerative diseases such as cancer, heart disease and diabetes.

The excessive demand for production of digestive enzymes is a consequence of our failure to take in sufficient quantity of raw food, for it is raw food only that supplies the food enzymes whose function it is to take the load off of the body's digestive enzymes. Dr. Howell tells us that any heat warm enough to feel uncomfortable to the hand is enough to injure enzymes in food. Enzyme destruction takes place at 116° F. The degree of enzyme destruction is a function of time and temperature. In the SAD, we cook almost everything we consume or it has already been cooked when we purchase it. Any pasteurized product (milk, juices) has been exposed to temperatures of approximately 145° and therefore is devoid of enzymes needed to help digest it. Pasteurization destroys the life force in enzymes. All processed foods have been exposed to heat by one means or another. Processed food therefore is not only short on vitamins and minerals, it is totally devoid of enzymes.

Many authorities in the field of nutrition recommend that the diet consist of anywhere between 50% and 100% raw food (the healthier we are, the more we can comfortably tolerate), with 70-80% being perhaps the most frequent recommendation. Once again, this is a dietary change that we advise to work into gradually, for an abrupt change will produce unpleasant symptoms as a result of the body's cleansing activities which are triggered by the raw foods. Including more raw foods in the diet enables the body to produce less concentrated digestive enzymes. If we all took in more exogenous enzymes (from the outside) in the form of raw foods, the body would not have to waste its enzyme potential on digesting foods. By raising our metabolic enzyme potential by increased intake of raw foods and/or enzyme supplements, we increase the body's ability to repair itself. It is the body's metabolic enzyme potential that is its mechanism for curing disease.

Man is the only animal that lives on an enzyme poor diet. A classic experiment done by Francis Pottenger, M.D. in 1946 dramatically illustrates the effects of such a diet. Dr. Pottenger took 900 cats and divided them into two groups - one was fed raw meat and milk, the other cooked meat and pasteurized milk. Over a ten year period, he found that each successive generation of cats fed cooked food showed an increase in degenerative diseases and other disorders common to man - arthritis, gastritis, liver atrophy, pyorrhea, loss of teeth and hair, osteoporosis, extreme irritability, kidney and thyroid disease, heart disease and cancer, etc. By the third generation all of these animals were sterile or congenitally malformed. Dr. Pottenger found that it took four generations to correct naturally the inherited damage caused by eating cooked food. None of the cats to whom he'd fed raw foods developed disease. They reproduced normally and lived to a ripe old age.

Cooked food digests much more slowly than raw food. This requires large amounts of energy. Ingestion of raw food conserves energy that can be redirected to rebuilding and repairing damaged tissue. Life span may be increased by increasing intake of raw foods, for in this manner our enzyme potential is conserved. It is not surprising to note that rats raised on raw food diets lived 30% longer than those raised on cooked foods.

Uncooked foods raise the microelectric potential throughout the body. The stronger the microelectric tensions, the better the ability of the body to repel toxic substances. All toxins are enzyme inhibitors. Sodium is an enzyme inhibitor. Potassium is an enzyme activator (Remember: We want to keep the potassium high and the sodium low in the cells to keep the electrical generators going). According to Georges Lakhovsky, eating cooked food physically destroys the oscillating circuit within the cell.

We recommend adding raw fruits and vegetables to the diet, while *slowly* reducing intake of the more concentrated foods. High protein diets are highly stimulatory and, if the body is accustomed to eating them in large amounts, it needs the stimulation they afford until such time as internal regulation can be restored. It may be that the vital force of the body is too depleted to tolerate raw foods initially. If so, start with cooked vegetables. In making the transition from the SAD to the optimal diet, it is imperative to go slowly, always adding before subtracting. Add the vegetables and whole grains. Cook them at first, and then, as your vitality level is raised, cook them only slightly and work your way into the introduction of totally raw foods, including fruit. Fruit should never be cooked. It becomes extremely acid forming. Many of us are so sick that abrupt transition to raw foods would cause a great deal of irritation to the intestines due to the excessive toxicity that is stirred up.

To retain enzyme activity in nuts and seeds, soak them overnight in purified or distilled water. The purpose of so doing is to release the 'enzyme inhibitors' which they contain. Nature supplies these foods with enzyme inhibitors to prevent them from germinating prematurely. It is contact with water (or moist soil) that triggers germination. The germination neutralizes or inactivates the enzyme inhibitors. When we soak our nuts and seeds we are encouraging germination and freeing up enzymes within the foods. Germinating and sprouting increases the enzyme content of foods six to twentyfold.

The squirrels in the wild know instinctively about enzyme activity - they bury their nuts. The contact with the moisture in the soil deactivates enzyme inhibitors through germination. By the time the squirrel digs up his nuts, they are digestable.

Considering the lack of enzymes in the SAD, it is not surprising that we spend over two billion dollars per year on digestive aids. Tagamet and Zantac (prescription drugs for gastrointestinal disorders) are now the top selling drugs in the country.

FAT

Fats in the diet consist of oils, butter, margarine and lard. All meats, of course, contain a relatively high percentage of fat, some much more than others. Nuts too have a high fat content, as do avocados. Fats are the most concentrated source of energy in the diet.

It is essential that we take in a certain amount of fat, for we cannot maintain health on a fat-free diet. Fats serve many vital functions: They facilitate oxygen transport; they lubricate and insulate muscles and organs, aid in the absorption of the fat soluble vitamins, nourish the skin, mucous membranes and nerves and help maintain body temperature. Fat, a certain amount of it in the diet, is essential. Nearly 40% of the SAD is composed of fat, however - that is at least double the amount needed to maintain good health.

There are basically two types of fat - saturated and

unsaturated. As the list below (from <u>Hydrogenation -</u> <u>America's Deadliest Killer</u>, p. 9) indicates, the saturated fats come primarily from animal sources, while the unsaturated ones come mainly from vegetable.

<u>Unsaturated</u>	<u>Saturated</u>
safflower oil	coconut oil
sunflower oil	all hydrogenated oils
olive oil	processed cheese
sesame oil	butter
soybean oil	pasteurized milk & cream
corn oil	all meat fats
peanut oil	poultry fats
cottonseed oil	
cod liver oil	
halibut liver oil	
avocado	
natural cheese	
all whole grains	
unpasteurized milk	

The unsaturated fats are generally found in liquid form, while the saturated ones are solid, usually hard at room temperature. Saturated fats have been implicated in the development of high cholesterol and consequently their reduction in the diet is frequently recommended. Nathan Pritikin points to a hamster study done by a Dr. Swank wherein five to six hours after consuming heavy cream these animals were found to have blockage of some 25% of their blood vessels, as well as a 1/3 reduction in the amount of oxygen in their blood. After a 72 hour fast, there was still a 5% deficit in blood oxygen level. Pritikin concludes that in the SAD "Where one fat meal follows another, everybody has blocked vessels all the time" ("Lipotoxemia: Nutrition and Degenerative Disease"). He notes that the American Heart Association recommends the substitution of unsaturated fats and contends with the efficacy of the recommendation based on the results of a 1965 study by Dr. Myer Friedman of Mt. Zion Hospital of San Francisco that was reported in the American Medical Association's journal. Dr. Friedman took forty firemen and photographed the fine vessels in their eyes after an overnight fast. All vessels were open. Five hours after drinking a glass of heavy cream, however, numerous blockages were seen in the vessels. Repeating the experiment using an unsaturated fat (safflower oil) in place of the saturated cream, resulted in blockages that were just as severe and numerous. The only difference was that at the end of nine hours, the saturated fat was out of the system and the unsaturated fat had not yet begun to leave. "One wonders", as Pritikin observed, "why the American Heart Association continues to endorse the use of unsaturated fats" ("Lipotoxemia: Nutrition and Degenerative Disease").

We contend that, in addition to considering saturated vs. unsaturated fats, it is imperative that we look at refined vs. unrefined, as well as pasteurized vs. unpasteurized in the effect of fat upon the body.

All vegetable oils are unsaturated. There is, however, a tremendous amount of difference between the effect of, say, refined safflower oil and that of unrefined. The refined version is processed with heat which destroys numerous nutrients, including lipase (the enzyme needed to break down fat), vitamin E (needed to help retard spoilage of the oil) and lecithin (needed to break down cholesterol). Refined oils, lacking these and other nutrients are incomplete foods, altered by man for commercial advantage. This alteration results in the elimination of nutrients essential to the proper utilization of the food. Elimination of the food enzyme, lipase, makes refined oils difficult to digest. This, coupled with the loss of lecithin needed to break down cholesterol, makes refined oil use a significant factor in today's high cholesterol epidemic, discussed more fully later in the chapter. A refined oil is not so labeled. The aisles of supermarkets are filled with refined vegetable oils. If stocked at all, the unrefined oils are generally kept in another section, usually a 'specialty' or 'health food' section. They may also be found in health food stores. Unrefined oils are labeled as such. Some may be labeled 'cold-pressed' or 'cold-processed'. 'Expellor pressed' may also appear on the label. While this method of expelling the oil is less destructive than the standard refining processes, it still does not produce a truly unrefined oil. Read your labels. And examine the oils. If they are light and crystal clear, they are refined.

We recommend that unrefined oils be used exclusively and that they be purchased in small quantities and kept in the refrigerator. The reason for this is that these oils oxidize or turn rancid very rapidly. Three factors cause oxidation - heat, light and air exposure. As soon as we remove the bottle cap, exposing the oil to air, a certain amount of oxidation takes place. Any time oils are used in cooking, of course, the heat produces rancidity, as does the heat produced at room temperature during storage. Oil does not have to smell bad to be rancid. The major problem with consumption of rancid oil is that it gives rise to the creation of free radicals. These are renegade chemical fragments which have been demonstrated to play a major causative role in degenerative disease development and in the aging process. Refrigeration of oils is vitally important. This is a fact not generally known, for it is not standard practice in homes, nor in restaurants, for oils to be refrigerated. Deep fat frying is particularly destructive, as extremely high temperatures are used. Many foods served in restaurants are so prepared and, if the restaurant is complying with health standards, the oil in the deep fat fryer may be changed only once a week.

We repeat the recommendation that only unrefined oils - and oil products - be used. This includes salad dressings, mayonnaise and peanut butter, all oil products that come in refined and unrefined form.

The body has a difficult time metabolizing fats (especially refined, saturated ones) if the liver is congested. And due to our eating habits, most of us have congested livers. Many of us function on only 30% or less of liver capacity due to depletion of the sodium in the organ to neutralize acid toxins in the body. The liver is the largest organ in the body and it performs a wide variety of functions, one of which is the manufacture of cholesterol. The cholesterol produced in our livers lubricates the artery walls and keeps the body from being washed away by its own blood currents. Although today's high cholesterol problem is synonymous with saturated fat consumption in the minds of most Americans, we believe that it is not saturated fats alone, but more importantly, the process of altering fats and creating unnatural, overheated fats that causes the cholesterol problem which brings us to the subject of

HYDROGENATION

'Saturated' and 'unsaturated' are chemical terms which refer to the way hydrogen is carried in the fatty acid molecule. Saturated fats contain extra bonds of hydrogen. Most fats contain a combination of saturated and unsaturated fatty acids. Foods, therefore, are not exclusively saturated or unsaturated, but primarily one or the other.

Hydrogenated or trans fats are man made. They do not spoil. Almost all processed foods today contain partially hydrogenated fats. Popular peanut butters which have a smooth, uniform texture and no oil floating on the top are an example. The jar of hydrogenated peanut butter you buy today will be just as 'fresh' 60 years from now as it was when it was packaged - and just as dangerous for you to consume.

The hydrogenation process was not created by, nor for, the food industry initially. In 1912 a French scientist, Paul Sabatier won the Nobel Prize for succeeding in hydrogenating organic compounds. He wasn't looking for a way to prolong shelf life in food, but rather for a way to make soap hard.

Sabatier succeeded in making the oil accept an extra

bond of hydrogen by using nickel as a catalyst. This same process is used in the hydrogenation of oils in the food industry. The fat, usually an unsaturated vegetable oil, is exposed to temperatures over 400° F. and small amounts of nickel are used to achieve the hydrogen bonding (see chapter 12 on toxic metals for information on the effect on the body), changing it from a liquid to a solid form. Margarine is an example of a hydrogenated fat. Margarine is generally thought to be unsaturated because it is made from vegetable oils which are unsaturated. However, once they have been through the hydrogenation process, they become super-saturated with hydrogen.

Once oil has gone through the process of hydrogenation, it is no longer an oil, but a plastic, a celluloid. Oils are <u>partially</u> hydrogenated, for were they completely hydrogenated, they would form into hard plastic-like chips. In the words of John H. Tobe, author of <u>Hydrogenation - America's Deadliest Killer</u> (p. 63):

Hydrogenated fat is nothing but sheer hard plastic, a new inorganic chemical compound that will not melt when you squeeze and rub it against your fingers, generating more than body heat. If these hydrogenated fats will not flow or at least break down at body temperatures, then exactly what would you expect your bloodstream to do with these plastic particles?

What your bloodstream does with these plastic particles is to retain them as obstructions to blood flow. They therefore become a significant factor in the incidence of coronary artery disease formation. It is no coincidence that heart disease increased with the introduction of hydrogenated fats in our diet. Homogenization is also a process which plays a significant role in heart disease and is discussed more fully in chapter 7. Remember the timetable: Americans were still fairly healthy in the first quarter of this century. Rapid decline in health followed the introduction of food refining processes, one of the most harmful of which is hydrogenation.

Hydrogenated oil, like mineral oil, prevents the absorption of fat-soluble vitamins (A, D, E, K) by binding with them in the body. Neither of these oils should be consumed, nor should mineral oil (baby oil) be rubbed on the skin, for it enters the bloodstream in that manner. Hydrogenated oils are devoid of natural fat emulsifiers; they inhibit proper gall bladder function and promote inflammation. Hydrogenated products include most commercial peanut butters, all margarines, shortenings and processed cheeses. And once again, they are an ingredient (though not necessarily appearing on the label) in most processed foods. We recommend the complete avoidance of hydrogenated fats. The body cannot process or utilize them. It is ironic that many people - even some doctors - feel that eating margarine is healthier than eating butter because they believe the margarine to be unsaturated. The truth, of course, is that the margarine is excessively saturated. Butter, especially in its raw state, with the lipase enzyme intact, is to be far preferred over margarine. Raw butter can be purchased in many health food stores, but note that it does have an expiration date, as it is made with raw, unpasteurized milk. (Chapter 7 contains a discussion of pasteurization and its effect upon food). Raw foods are generally to be preferred over cooked ones (and pasteurization is a form of cooking), for they are whole foods, with their enzymes intact. The lipase enzyme which breaks down fat is not found in pasteurized milk, butter or cheese, but is present in these foods in their raw state. The American public consumes copious amounts of pasteurized dairy products. These products, lacking in the protease and lipase enzymes (needed to break down proteins and fats), are not properly digested and result in putre-faction (and subsequent creation of acid toxins), as well as elevated triglyceride (blood fat) and choles-terol (arterial fat) levels in the body.

Hydrogenated fats are entirely synthetic and their production creates abnormal fatty acids, the next subject of discussion.

When fats are eaten, they're broken down into glycerin and fatty acids (also known as vitamin F). Even if no fat is eaten, the body can make most of these fats from sugars. But three of them it cannot: **linoleic, linolenic** and **arachidonic** acid. These are the Essential Fatty Acids (EFAs).

Animal studies show that EFA deficiencies result in eczema and sterility. Overweight too is linked with too *little* fat consumption, as Adelle Davis explains in Let's Eat Right to Keep Fit (p.45):

For three reasons, eating too little fat is probably a major cause of overweight. First, many seemingly fat persons are only waterlogged; an adequate diet including salad dressing daily often causes them to lose pounds. Second, it has been proved by what is known as the respiratory quotient that when the essential fatty acids are insufficiently supplied, the body changes sugar to fat much more rapidly than is normal; Dr. Bloor points out that it would seem as if the body were speedily trying to produce the missing nutrients. This quick change makes the blood sugar plunge downward, causing you to be as starved as a wolf; the chances are that you overeat and gain weight. Third, fats are more satisfying than any other foods. If you forego eating 100 calories of fat per meal, you usually become so hungry that you eat 500 calories of starch and/or sugar simply because you cannot resist them; unwanted pounds creep on.

In theory, arachidonic acid and linolenic acid can be synthesized from linoleic acid *if* it is sufficiently supplied in the diet:

Linoleic ▶ Arachidonic
▼
Linolenic (or Gamma Linolenic Acid - GLA)

However, the processing of oils renders linoleic acid inactive so that it cannot be converted to GLA. Other factors also prevent this conversion: nutrient deficiencies (B6, zinc, magnesium), viral infection, aging, high intake of fat and/or alcohol.

Linoleic acid comes primarily from the seeds of vegetables, linolenic acid or GLA from the leaves and arachidonic acid, also known as Omega 6, comes primarily from animal sources except fish. Fish provide another fatty acid, eicosapentaenoic acid (EPA), also known as Omega 3. Omega 3 can also be produced from GLA:

Linoleic (from seeds) ▶ Arachidonic (Omega 6 from animals, except fish)

Linolenic (or GLA from leaves) ▶ EPA (Omega 3 from fish)

Since the bulk of the SAD is composed of animal products and most of the oils we take in are from the seeds rather than the leaves of plants, it can readily be seen how EPA deficiencies can develop, as they have in this country in recent years. Without being able to make that conversion from linoleic to linolenic acid and subsequently to EPA, Americans are facing an EPA deficiency unless they find a way to take in more EPA. Taking in larger quantities of fish or fish oil is one way. It is a way that has been touted as a cure for the cholesterol problem. The apparent beneficial effect of fish oil in the SAD can be attributed to the fact that it is helping to restore a balance of fatty acids. The widespread imbalance of which we speak looks like this:

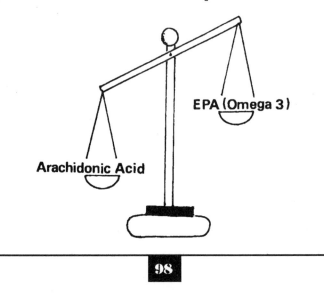

It is estimated that Americans take in ten to twenty times more arachidonic acid than EPA. This excessive intake of arachidonic acid is due primarily to high meat consumption. The lack of EPA in the SAD is also attributable to the fact that <u>Omega 3 is removed from processed foods</u> because it causes them to become rancid rapidly.

The imbalance of fatty acids illustrated on page 98 results in an imbalance or overproduction of prostaglandins. A prostaglandin is a powerful, hormone-like regulator which may affect many of the body's systems, including the immune system. Prostaglandins live about one second and are produced in the body when and where they are needed. They are involved in such processes as blood clotting, inflammation, pain perception and smooth muscle contraction. What they do depends upon the <u>balance</u> of fatty acids. This balance is thrown off with the absence of sufficient quantities of EPA in the diet. The hydrogenation of fats also intensifies EPA deficiencies and produces 'weird' prostaglandins.

It has been demonstrated that EPA reduces triglycerides and increases the amount of HDL ('good' cholesterol) in the blood. We should certainly be concerned about getting sufficient quantities of this fatty acid in our diet. We do not, however, recommend the taking of fish oil, nor the excessive consumption of fish. The dangers of overconsumption of protein, especially animal protein, have already been addressed. As far as fish oil is concerned, the SAD already contains too much oil in general. And anytime we separate the oil from the whole food, we are asking for trouble, whether the oil came from vegetable or animal sources. All such extracted oils oxidize very rapidly, as was already mentioned. We therefore recommend that, rather than turning to fish as a source of EPA, you consider the following rich sources of the fatty acid: flax seed, linseed oil, fresh green leafy vegetables, sea vegetables, nuts, seeds, borage, black currents, soybeans, olive oil and evening primrose oil. If you must cook with oil, olive oil is one of the most stable and heat resistant of the oils. Peanut oil, sesame and canola oil are also more heat resistant than the lighter oils such as safflower.

Three of the B vitamins - choline, inositol and vitamin B6 - help maintain normal blood cholesterol levels. Choline and inositol, along with fat and EFAs, are components of lecithin, a substance manufactured in the body which breaks down cholesterol. It cannot be adequately manufactured, however, in the absence of vitamin B complex rich foods in the diet. We have already discussed how food processing (particularly the milling of grains) results in widespread B complex deficiencies.

It has been demonstrated that "experimental high blood cholesterol cannot be produced by feeding cholesterol and saturated fats if even a minimal amount of lecithin is included in the diet" (Adelle Davis, Let's Eat Right to Keep Fit, p. 118). Lecithin then is essential to cholesterol reduction. You will recall that it is one of the substances that is removed from oils when they are refined. It is established that experimental arteriosclerosis can be prevented by giving choline, inositol and the EFAs (or lecithin which supplies them).

Richard Passwater tells us "evidence shows that high fat consumption when accompanied by plenty of the essential nutrients which all cells need does not cause atherosclerosis."

It has been found too that fiber lowers cholesterol - hence the craze to down as much oat bran as possible. Please remember that bran comes from the whole grain, but is discarded in the milling process. Were we eating the whole grain in the first place, we would not have the need for the additional bran. Consumed by itself, bran can be an irritant to the intestines. It is highly stimulatory when consumed apart from the rest of the grain and should not be ingested in that manner in large quantities.

It is important to recognize that, while no cholesterol is found in foods of vegetable origin, many vegetable fats are more saturated either by nature or by hydrogenation than are animal fats. These saturated fats (coconut oil, margarine, shortenings, processed cheeses and peanut butter) *increase the blood cholesterol by increasing the need for choline.*

Blood cholesterol does not travel through the body on its own, but must attach itself to a solid structure in the bloodstream. In humans cholesterol binds with lipoproteins - high density (HDL) and low density (LDL). The HDL contains less cholesterol, more protein. It is composed principally of lecithin and is known as the 'good' cholesterol. LDL's function is to supply the cells of the arterial walls with some of the cholesterol they need. This is a vital function, so LDL is not truly a 'bad' cholesterol. It is only bad when it is excessively produced.

Bear in mind that cholesterol is a lubricant that keeps the blood oily so it can flow freely. It tends to clog up the arteries, however, if the walls have built up deposits of inorganic minerals. Cholesterol can collect in this case, for the inorganic mineral deposits offer another solid substance to which the blood cholesterol might attach itself. Sources of inorganic minerals include certain mineral supplements, enriched foods, pasteurized products and hard water (see next chapter).

In summation then, one wishing to lower his cholesterol might wish to:

... avoid processed, refined oils, use only unrefined
... avoid completely all hydrogenated fats
... increase intake of EPA through natural, non-animal sources
... avoid intake of inorganic minerals
... avoid homogenized products
... increase intake of lecithin
... assure intake of sufficient lipase by using raw fat products
... avoid pasteurized dairy products
... increase fiber intake (fresh fruits, vegetables, whole grains)
... decrease sugar consumption (see next page)

CARBOHYDRATES

All the plants we eat, whether fruits, vegetables or grains are carbohydrates. Sugars and starches are included in this category. The body converts all sugars and starches to glucose (blood sugar). You will recall that ATP (the fuel for the electrical generator, the sodium/potassium pump) is made up primarily of glucose and oxygen. Of all of the nutrients, carbohydrates are the best source of glucose. They are the chief source of energy for all body functions and muscular exertion, providing us with immediately available calories for energy by producing heat in the body when carbon in the system unites with oxygen in the bloodstream.

Carbohydrates can be manufactured in the body from some amino acids and the glycerol component of fats. Therefore, there is no established RDA. Carbohydrates are necessary to assist in the digestion and assimilation of other foods. Those found in fruits and vegetables help reduce the need for protein.

As we have previously stated, refined grains have had their fiber and germ and many of their vitamins and minerals removed. Some, but not all of the B vitamins removed during milling, are replaced in the 'enriching' process. B vitamin deficiencies are therefore created as a result of the widespread use of refined carbohydrates. If the B vitamins are absent, carbohydrate combustion cannot take place and indigestion and symptoms of nausea and heartburn occur. Americans take in large quantities of refined carbohydrates and cannot properly digest them, not only because of B vitamin deficiencies, but also due to improperly combined foods. A cardinal rule of food combining is to avoid eating starchy carbohydrates at the same meal with proteins. Combinations like cheese and bread, milk and cereal, potatoes and meat and eggs and toast are as American as apple pie - and just as difficult to digest! Proteins require an acid digestive secretion, while carbohydrates call for an alkaline one. We all know what happens when acid meets alkaline - the fluids become neutralized and nothing gets digested. The protein putrifies. The carbohydrate ferments. This means they rot in the body, creating toxins which are acid in nature.

The SAD is composed of approximately 40% carbohydrate foods (largely refined ones). We would do well to double this percentage (achieved by reducing fats and proteins), consuming exclusively **unrefined** carbohydrates - i.e., whole grain products, fresh fruits and vegetables. Considering the prevalence of blood sugar disorders today, it would also be advisable for us to increase the amount of complex carbohydrates in our diet. These consist of starches, vegetables and legumes. Unrefined complex carbohydrates take longer to digest than refined ones or simple sugars and therefore help the pancreas to keep the blood sugar stable. Simple sugars include sucrose and other concentrated sweeteners, such as honey, molasses, maple syrup. Fruits may also be placed in this category, as they require little breakdown in the body and are digested very rapidly. Although they are in many ways the ideal food for the body, the ideal diet can only be handled by the perfectly healthy body, and there are some fruits (citrus in particular) which most of us are not yet healthy enough to consume, for they would cause too severe a cleansing reaction in a toxin laden body. Table sugar requires some digestive action, but is not nearly so complex as starches which require prolonged enzymatic action in order to be broken down into glucose. Increasing complex carbohydrates also increases fiber in the diet, needed for good bowel action.

In order for the whole system to be at its best, there must be a balance between the glucose and oxygen. When this balance is off the body goes into a state of stress, with a resulting strain on the endocrine system, leading to glandular exhaustion. All sugars provide glucose to the body. However, some are more usable than others, are more assimilable. All man-made sugars - those extracted and concentrated from food sources and those made from chemicals - are difficult for the body to utilize. While they provide abundant glucose, they are lacking in the nutrients needed to utilize the glucose. What follows is one of the most comprehensive listings of sugars and other sweeteners we have found. This information is from Earl Mindell's <u>Unsafe at Any Meal</u>:

SUCROSE - table sugar. A disaccharide (double sugar - glucose + fructose). It has no nutrients, requires B vitamins to assimilate, comes from cane or beet sugar.

GLUCOSE - the body's blood sugar. A monosaccharide, found in most fruits. It is readily assimilated by the body.

DEXTROSE - made from cornstarch. It is a monosaccharide which is chemically identical to glucose.

FRUCTOSE - (levulose) Found in fruits, but many fruits are mainly sucrose. It is absorbed more slowly than sucrose, is highly refined and devoid of nutrients, even when derived from natural sources.

MALTOSE - a non-nutritious disaccharide made from the malting of grains.

LACTOSE - Glucose + galactose. It is as non-nutritive as all other refined sugars, but it feeds the beneficial intestinal bacteria.

BROWN SUGAR - white, refined sugar with molasses coloring.

RAW or TURBINADO SUGAR - is packaged at 96% sucrose (table sugar is 99%) and has no nutritive benefit.

BLACKSTRAP MOLASSES - the liquid that remains after beet and cane sugar have been thoroughly processed and the sucrose has been removed. It is still 65% sucrose and contains minor, but useful amounts of iron, calcium, potassium and B vitamins. The darker the molasses, the more nutritious.

HONEY - has the highest sugar content of all sweeteners (65 calories per teaspoon as compared to refined sugar's 48). It has small amounts of potassium, calcium and phosphorus and contains natural enzymes and pollen IF unheated. Some varieties have been found to contain carcinogens that the bees have extracted from flowers sprayed with cancer-causing chemicals. Some bees are fed sugar.

MAPLE SYRUP - 65% sucrose. In commercial preparation, sap may be gathered in lead-soldered buckets and formaldehyde pellets used to keep the tap holes from healing and to increase the sap flow. Chemical anti-foaming agents are sometimes used.

MALT SYRUPS - made from several grains, they contain mainly maltose and glucose. They are nutritionally superior, but not as sweet as maple syrups. Some have added sweetness from commercial CORN SYRUP which is industrially refined glucose. Barley malt syrup is the least sweet, but the most wholesome. These syrups are usually not made from organic grains.

XYLITOL - Although found naturally in berries, fruits and mushrooms, it is generally extracted from birch cellulose. It is considered a carbohydrate alcohol and has some value as sugar, but is metabolized differently. Large doses in long term feeding studies have caused tumors and organ injury in animals. Used in IVs, it has caused liver, kidney and brain disturbances in humans.

SORBITOL - half as sweet as sucrose. It occurs naturally in fruits, berries, algae and seaweeds. It is made industrially from hydrogen and commercial glucose (corn syrup). It is absorbed slowly and large doses have a laxative effect.

MANNITOL - occurs naturally in beets, celery, olives, but is made commercially in the same was as sorbitol. It is half as sweet as sugar and produces diarrhea at lower levels than does sorbitol.

ASPARTAME (Nutrasweet and Equal) - composed of two amino acids, phenylalinine and aspartic acid, it is 200 times sweeter than sugar, though it has the same amount of calories. Its use has been implicated in numerous disorders ranging from nausea and headaches to seizures, rashes, blindness and brain damage.

SACCHARIN - a non-caloric petroleum derivative, it is 300 - 500 times sweeter than sugar. It is not absorbed by the body, but has been linked with bladder cancer in laboratory animals.

CYCLAMATE - a non-caloric sweetener, 30 times sweeter than sugar, it has been implicated in causing testicular atrophy and chromosome damage. It has been banned in the U.S. and in Britain.

These last three, aspartame, saccharin and cyclamate are totally man-made. Another sweetener is an herbal one, stevia. It is 30 to 40 times sweeter than sugar and is said to have no harmful effects. As you can see, there are drawbacks in the use of any of the sweeteners listed by Mindell. Our best source of glucose is whole foods, preferably organically grown ones. Mineral rich fruits and vegetables are very sweet tasting. Those grown on impoverished soils have a bitter taste. Grain sprouted to 1" in length is as sweet as candy. We would do well to eliminate or significantly decrease our use of exogenous sweeteners. They are too rich for the body.

The word 'sugar' as used henceforth in this chapter will refer to sucrose. Sucrose is cane or beet sugar. It is the refined, white table sugar with which we are all too familiar. As Dr. Mindell notes, it contains no nutrients (except calories) and requires B vitamins to assimilate. So, sugar consumption makes extra demands on the body's already depleted supply of B vitamins (see chapter 8). In 1870 Americans consumed 11 teaspoons of sugar daily. A hundred years later, in 1970, we were taking in 32 teaspoons, an almost threefold increase. In 1980, the rate of sugar consumption was up to 38 teaspoons per person per day. In 1978 we took in 128 lbs. per person annually (over 40 t.), with only 6% of that intake coming from natural sources. Where are we getting all of this sugar? Much of it is hidden in our food. Start reading labels. There are almost 100 different kinds of sugar listed on them. Know that anything ending in 'ose' is some form of sugar.

There are many harmful effects of overconsumption of sugar. It appears to derange the apestat mechanism so that the body's inherent wisdom regarding food selection becomes impaired. We then build addictive patterns, craving more sugar, rather than needed nutrients. Sugar displaces other foods in the sense that it occupies space which could otherwise be filled with nutritious foods. As already mentioned, it robs the body of B vitamins needed to metabolize it. It also destroys vitamin C and has been linked with a build up of cholesterol in the blood. It has been found that people with moderately severe atherosclerosis usually have mild hypoglycemia and those with moderate and severe diabetes have especially severe atherosclerosis. In other words, the worse the blood sugar disorder, the higher the cholesterol count. It has been demonstrated that many diabetics have more than ample amounts of insulin in their blood. According to Pritikin, it is the presence of excessive levels of fat that prevents the insulin from getting into the cell system. Since life begins and ends at the cellular level, unless we can get nutrients into the cells where they belong, they will not nourish the body. Blood sugar disorders themselves are, in part, a consequence of overconsumption of sugar. Excess sugar intake also leads to increased urinary excretion of calcium, contributing to deficiency of this mineral. And lastly, sugar is acid forming. Intake of large amounts contributes to the creation of acidosis in the system, with subsequent demineralization of muscles, organs and bones to buffer the acid if the needed alkaline minerals are not supplied in the diet.

BLOOD SUGAR DISORDERS

The brain uses 50% of all available glucose in the blood. Changes in blood sugar level affect the brain and therefore affect behavior.

Most of us know that diabetes is a condition of too much sugar in the blood (hyperglycemia) and not enough insulin (hypoinsulinism). Insulin is the hormone that makes it possible for glucose to enter the cells and be converted into energy. Each time that we consume sugar, the pancreas is called upon to secrete insulin. That insulin will drive about 30% of the sugar consumed into the cells. The other 70% is stored in the liver as glycogen.

Insulin supplementation (oral or injectable) is the medical treatment of choice for diabetes. The exogenous insulin forces the cell to accept glucose and sugar levels are thereby controlled. Insulin supplementation is by no means a cure for diabetes, however.

To better understand diabetes, we need to look at the mechanism of action of its precursor, hypoglycemia (low blood sugar). At first glance, it would seem that diabetes and low blood sugar are opposites, for one involves too much sugar in the blood, the other too little. In reality, however, hypoglycemia precedes diabetes. It was first identified in 1924 when Dr. Seal Harris noticed non-diabetics who were showing signs of insulin shock: nervousness, tiredness, cold sweats, convulsions, fainting. The standard test for measuring blood sugar levels at that time called for blood to be analyzed at hourly intervals for three consecutive hours after a fasting patient was given glucose orally. By extending this test up to six hours, Dr. Harris found that patients who may have shown normal (80-120) readings initially would often experience a drop in the blood sugar level in the final hours of the test. When the blood sugar level fell below 80, the condition was termed 'hypoglycemia'. It was further found through this extended glucose tolerance test that some patients who showed blood sugar levels above normal initially (in the diabetic range) would dip into the hypoglycemic range in the final hours of the test. This condition was termed 'dysinsulinism'. It is best treated in the same manner as hypoglycemia. Since the condition cannot be detected with the standard test and such a test is likely to yield false results, it could result in a patient with dysinsulinism being misdiagnosed as diabetic. Administration of insulin to such a patient would certainly create problems, for when he is in his hypoglycemic phase, his body is already producing too much insulin. To clarify, let's look at the terms:

HYPOglycemia = HYPERinsulinism = Low Blood Sugar

HYPERglycemia = HYPOinsulinism = High Blood Sugar (Diabetes)

To better understand the causal relationship between these apparently opposite conditions, let us consider what happens when we eat. When we take in sugar and/or caffeine and alcohol, the pancreas secretes insulin. When we consume these items frequently in large quantities, we are making rather tall demands upon the pancreas. It is therefore kept quite busy secreting insulin and after a time goes into hyperactivity. When the pancreas secretes <u>too much</u> insulin, we have a condition of too little sugar in the blood. Now, remember the sugar that was originally stored in the liver as glycogen? When the blood sugar level begins to drop during periods when we are not eating, it is the job of the liver to convert some of this glycogen back into sugar to be supplied to the blood to raise the blood sugar level. However, as has been previously discussed, most of us have impaired liver function. When the blood sugar level starts to drop, the hypothalamus, whose job it is to monitor internal body functions, directs the adrenal glands to secrete adrenalin or epinepherine which triggers the liver to convert its glycogen to sugar. This is what is supposed to happen. A breakdown in communications between these organs, as well as a liver impairment can result in hypoglycemia going unchecked, however. So, low blood sugar has a lot to do with the liver, not just the pancreas. Most people today, certainly those on the SAD are hypoglycemic, but just don't know it. And hypoglycemia is the first step toward diabetes. Remember: An organ goes first into **hyper**function and then into **hypo**function. Over a period of time, the overworked pancreas may indeed decrease its insulin production, at which time we have adult onset diabetes. Diabetes is the result of a severely dysfunctional pancreas. But remember too what Pritikin pointed out: Many diabetics have sufficient insulin in their blood; it is simply not getting to the cellular level due to obstruction by fatty deposits. Pritikin gave examples of diabetics whose condition improved significantly after eliminating fat from their diets. The link between high cholesterol and blood sugar disorders is well established.

Sub-clinical hypoglycemia can produce such symptoms as irritability, anxiety, unstable temper, moodi-

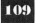

ness, headache and fatigue - a familiar set of symptoms, often misdiagnosed. Hypoglycemia is an underlying condition in asthma, allergies, hay fever, rheumatic fever, ulcers and in most cases of mental illness.

The standard medical treatment for hypoglycemia is dietary control, with recommendation of frequent ingestion of high protein foods. This may make us feel better, due to the stimulation provided by the protein, but we'll be getting worse all the while. While exogenous protein can be converted into glucose, it is not the best source and, as has already been demonstrated, a high protein diet causes putrefaction in the colon and production of poisonous byproducts that cause trapped plasma protein.

For the hypoglycemic we recommend a diet that is low in sugar (with **no** refined sugar), high in complex, unrefined carbohydrates and low in animal protein. Such a diet can be based on three food groups: (1) grains, seeds and nuts (2) vegetables and (3) fruits. It would be well to avoid the sweet fruits, also citrus, for the latter is an aggressive cleanser, too strong for most of us to tolerate. All vegetables and their juices (fresh, raw juices) are excellent to rebuild the body. Carrot juice is especially beneficial in hypoglycemia. While more food value is derived from grains that are sprouted than those that are cooked, the hypoglycemic will do well initially to cook his grains, for the cooked grains digest twice as slowly as the raw ones, releasing their sugar into the blood gradually during as much as 6-8 hours after a meal. Whole grains play a key role in the diet, for B vitamins (which they supply) are essential to the control of blood sugar level. Salt is to be avoided, for too much causes a loss of blood potassium which leads to a drop in blood sugar.

Chromium is also needed to metabolize the blood sugar. It works with insulin, facilitating the entry of glucose into the cells. Without chromium, the **tissues become insensitive to insulin**. The lower the total body chromium level gets, the worse the glucose metabolism functions. White sugar in the diet contributes to the loss of chromium from the body and consequent deficiency. Pure chromium is poorly absorbed by the body which produces its own in a special molecular structure called GTF (Glucose Tolerance Factor) made up of cysteine, glycine, glutamic acid, niacin and chromium. Yeast is an excellent source of GTF, but is contraindicated for patients with candida albicans. Brewer's yeast is popular in health circles. However, it is cooked and therefore a dead food. Baker's yeast is preferred. It is a vegetable without a cellulose wall. It is nutritious and well tolerated when consumed by itself in a glass of water. Mixed with fruit or fruit juice it ferments, causing gastric upset.

Dr. William Philpot in Brain Allergies has observed that food allergies, gone long undetected, can produce behavioral abnormalities, even psychoses. He has developed methods of identifying food allergens and has found that any food, regardless of glucose content, to which a person is allergic can cause a disturbance in blood sugar level. Food and environmental allergies have become widespread. The allergic reaction is an auto-immune response which ironically can be attributed, at least in part, to the use of allopathic medicines, particularly antibiotics. Dr. Reckeweg (Homotoxicology) tells us that molecules of the drug, along with molecules of the bacterial endotoxins (from the remains of dead micro-organisms), become encoded in the body's own protein and the immune response is therefore launched against self, as well as non-self.

In summary then, the increased intake of unrefined, complex carbohydrates, the avoidance of hydrogenated fats and the gradual introduction of raw foods into the diet is recommended. Where fats are concerned, small amounts of unrefined oils are essential to the body. In their extracted form these oils oxidize (turn rancid) rapidly and therefore should be used with discretion. Extracted oils - both of the saturated and unsaturated variety - can be a burden to the body, especially if they are refined and therefore lacking in the enzymes needed to digest them. With oils, as with all other food products, it is most desirable that they be consumed as an integral part of the whole food.

The diet can more closely approximate the ideal as alkaline reserve and vitality are restored to the body. Whether we are dealing with hypoglycemia, diabetes, heart disease, cancer or arthritis the road to reversal of the degenerative disease process is the same. Violation of nature's laws can result in a myriad of conditions, but restoration of health is achieved by obedience to those laws, which remain constant regardless of the variety of symptoms expressed.

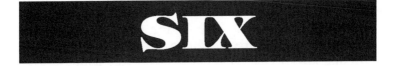

WATER

Water is the most abundant and important nutrient in the body. The average person can go five weeks without food, but only five days without water. It is a nutrient that serves many vital functions in the body: it is a carrier for oxygen, other nutrients and metabolic waste products, helping to flush toxins out of the system; it is a chief constituent of protoplasm, 90% of the blood being made up of water; it is required for the enzymatic activity of all metabolic processes and pure water is the primary solvent in the body, dissolving substances so that they can be assimilated or taken in by every cell.

Up to 70% of the body is composed of water. What percentage of our diet then would you think should be made up of water? - about 70%, according to many authorities. The high water content foods once again are fruits, vegetables and sprouts. These will also have the advantage of helping to alkalize the system and providing fiber for the intestines. If 70% of our diet IS made up of high water content foods, we won't need to worry about our exogenous intake of water. However, the SAD is composed primarily of concentrated foods with little to no water content. When partaking of such a diet, large volumes of water must be consumed to replenish the nutrients in the bloodstream and to activate the kidneys so they'll be able to get rid of the excess poisonous by-products. Americans are not big water drinkers - in fact, we consume more soft drinks than we do water! Insufficient intake of water causes incomplete elimination - and remember: Elimination is one of the four basic elements in the C.A.R.E. model. Inadequate elimination can adversely affect the other three processes (circulation, assimilation and relaxation), resulting in a build up of toxic accumulations.

If we are consuming a diet high in fruits, vegetables and sprouts and are therefore not thirsty, then there is no need to force 6 - 8 glasses or more of water per day into the body. Too much water will eventually damage the kidneys and cause further disease. It can waterlog the tissues, impair cellular function and lower the capacity of the blood to absorb and carry oxygen. For the person on the SAD, we would recommend intake of 1/2 oz. of water per lb. of body weight. Soft drinks are not a viable substitute, nor is coffee, tea or pasteurized juice. *Fresh* fruits and vegetable juices, on the other hand, are composed largely of naturally distilled water, which will satisfy the needs of the body.

Drinking a glass of water first thing in the morning (room temperature pure water) will provide moisture for the intestines and help keep the bowels regular.

Water leaves the stomach very rapidly - in about five minutes - if consumed alone. Ingesting water at mealtime is to be avoided, as it will result in dilution of digestive juices.

One final word of advice: If you are on the SAD and therefore taking in large quantities of water, take them in a little at a time - 4 oz. at once, rather than guzzling down three times that amount and overworking the kidneys.

Once we have made the basic and necessary changes in our diet, the quantity of exogenous water taken into the system need not be an issue. All of us, however, need to be concerned with the *quality* of water that we consume, our next topic of discussion.

WATER QUALITY

Only 1% of the world's water is drinkable. The rest is sea water or ice. This being the case, it is critically important that we guard this precious 1% against contamination. We don't seem to be doing such a good job of this, as our own Public Health Service tells us that <u>several million Americans</u> are drinking water that is potentially hazardous, contaminated with bacteria and chemicals.

Those of us on the public water system may choose to believe that our water is safe to drink because all the 'bad stuff' was filtered out at the municipal water treatment plant, but this is not so. Only suspended matter (silt, sand, etc.) can be mechanically filtered out. The filtered water still has sediment, micro-organisms and dissolved chemicals. Even if the water *were* safe when it left the plant, there is no guarantee that it would be safe when it entered your home, for faulty pipes and soldering leaks can cause contamination. The fact of the matter is that tap water is *not* pure. In some cities it has been used as many as five times by other people before it reaches your home!

More than 700 different chemicals have been identified in American drinking water to date. The Environmental Protection Agency (E.P.A.) tells us that our communities' water supplies are "liberally laced with asbestos, pesticides, heavy metals like lead and cadmium, arsenic, nitrates, sodium and a variety of chemicals that are known carcinogens" (<u>Dr. Donsbach</u> <u>Tells You What You Always Wanted to Know About</u> <u>Water</u>, p.12). The pollution problem has become so all pervasive that traces of DDT have been found in the ice at the North Pole! The U.S. General Accounting Office in a 3/3/82 report to the administrator of the E.P.A. reported: "The safe drinking water act of 1974 represents the first national commitment to provide safe drinking water. Yet, during fiscal year 1980, over 146,000 violations of the drinking water regulations were recorded against community water systems."

Chemical pollution has also reached ground water (via seepage from landfills into aquafers, ruptured underground fuel oil storage tanks and septic tanks), resulting in the contamination of wells. Once contaminated, groundwater can remain so for hundreds of thousands of years. The chances of contamination are good when we consider that 8 out of 10 Americans live near a toxic waste dump or source. Micro-organisms, linked with infectious disease can and have been transmitted through the water supply.

In many communities, water has become so polluted that it can only be made safe to drink by loading it with chlorine to kill the parasites, viruses, bacteria, algae, yeasts and molds. (Chlorine is a potent chemical used in World War II to kill *people*.) Ironically, the chlorination process itself creates carcinogens. When it combines with other pollutants or even with natural organic matter, such as decaying vegetation, it forms new compounds known as trihalomethanes (ThMs). ThMs consist of such deadly chemicals as chloroform and bromoform and carbon tetrachloride. Dr. Kurt Donsbach links the high incidence of kidney, bladder and urinary tract cancer in New Orleans with the fact that the water there is chlorinated in excess of government standards to guard against disease. The result is the creation of 66 new carcinogenic compounds. It is also interesting that when chlorine combines with animal fat, it forms a sticky, pastelike substance that adheres to arterial walls. ThMs are a known causative agent in atherosclerosis, as are cadmium and fluoride, also found in tap water. Recent studies have shown evidence that links chlorination to increased incidences of colon and rectal cancer.

Some people believe that boiling water will make it safe to drink. This is not so, for boiling may actually concentrate some contaminants, such as fluorides. If you *must* drink polluted water, however, boil it for at least ten minutes. This will at least kill some of the bacteria. It will not, however, remove the inorganic minerals, nor the dissolved solids and many of the chemicals.

If boiling water doesn't purify it, where can we turn for pure water - to rain water, to bottled water? When rainwater falls through the air, it picks up the bacteria, dust, smoke, chemicals and minerals in it, so that the water is no longer pure by the time it falls to earth. As far as bottled water is concerned, the standards for it are the same as for municipal water systems. It is of extremely variable quality. Although bottled water is regulated by the FDA as food, bottlers of water are not required to disclose their water sources.

Perhaps our best pure water source is the water found in fruits and vegetables. It is distilled by nature. The distilling process turns water into vapor and, through condensation, back again into pure water. Electric distillers do the same thing, but most do not remove the ThMs . They are also costly to operate - up to 20¢ per gallon. Distillation does, however, remove inorganic minerals from the water and this is desirable. Inorganic mineral deposits can be created by boiling tap water in a kettle. After a time, a hard scale will build up on the inside of the vessel. When we consume tap water, the same thing happens in our body. Inorganic minerals, not usable by the body, form deposits in various locations. They may be laid down in the joints, in which case we call it arthritis. Found in the intestines, these deposits cause constipation. In the kidneys or gall bladder they form stones; in the ears, deafness; in the arteries, atherosclerosis, etc.

Now, while tap water lays down these inorganic mineral deposits which the body cannot assimilate, distilled or purified water, which is devoid of inorganic minerals, will actually help dissolve these undesirable deposits. It will not remove the body's vital organic minerals, however. These stay in the tissues where they belong. Once these inorganic mineral deposits have been dissolved, gentle massage can assist in directing them out of the body through the lymphatic system.

Medical science does not acknowledge the presence of

inorganic mineral deposits in the body as a causative factor in disease. However, were it not for the presence of calcium deposits along artery walls, the outline of arteries would never show up on x-rays. These deposits, Dr. Allen E. Banik (The Choice is Clear) tells us, give cholesterol something else to cling to. He also informs us that hard water seals each cell with a film so that oxygen cannot reach the imprisoned cell. Nature then develops new cells which thrive on less oxygen - cancer cells.

So, when we speak of pure water, we refer to water that is not only devoid of pollutants, but of minerals as well. Let's look at some water purification techniques commonly used:

WATER PURIFICATION

Many people believe that water softeners remove the hard minerals. Actually, nothing is removed; the hard mineral ions are simply altered, with calcium and magnesium being replaced with sodium. Soft water is therefore high in sodium. Water softeners do not filter out micro-organisms and other pollutants. Such water is not recommended for drinking purposes.

We maintain that the best purification units combine a pre-filter, carbon filter and a Reverse Osmosis (RO) membrane. A pre-filter is actually a sediment filter used to remove undissolved solids. It traps large particles and heavy sediment. A carbon filter removes organic pollutants and chlorine, as well as some pesticides, but not most minerals. The 'activated' form of carbon or charcoal has been fired to a high temperature in the absence of oxygen. This process creates millions of microscopic pores that can trap particles. Others become stuck to its surface or *ad*sorbed. A granulated, activated carbon filter used in conjunction with an RO system will effectively remove chlorine and ThMs. Carbon filters are also useful in eradicating unpleasant tastes and odors. These filters need to be changed often (roughly every six months, more or less, depending upon the size and flow requirements). If not replaced at regular intervals, they can become clogged with pollutants, or worse yet, when the carbon is used up, the previously filtered pollutants may be allowed to flow back into the water. Clogged carbon filters can also become a breeding ground for bacteria. Many carbon filter home units run the water through in seconds and the consumer is led to believe that he has instantly pure water. This is not possible, for it takes 7 - 18 minutes to trap many cancer-causing solvents. We believe that the carbon filter is useful as a back up filtration system, but would turn to the RO membrane as the primary filtering mechanism for drinking water. A shower filter for removing chlorine is also desirable.

The first RO units were made in the early 50s by the U.S. Department of Interior for the desalinization of salt water. RO is a process by which water is forced through a semi-permeable membrane which separates the pure water from pollutants. The RO membrane removes inorganics, viruses, bacteria, pesticides, detergents, asbestos, heavy metals, sodium salts and nuclear contaminants. These units are inexpensive to operate, costing about 10 cents per gallon. No electricity is used. The units attach directly to the faucet and most have a built in holding tank for the treated water. They do not produce pure water instantly, for it takes time for the water to trickle through the microscopic pores of the RO membrane. How much time depends on the individual unit. An RO membrane does not last forever, but does not need to be replaced as frequently as the carbon filter. It should be checked periodically (through water analysis) and can be expected to last 2-3 years. There are many companies producing RO units. There are also several producing units which combine a pre-filter, carbon filter and RO membrane which we find to be a desirable combination. RO and distillation are the only two methods of purification that produce extremely pure water--i.e., water devoid of minerals and most other Total Dissolved Solids (TDS). Purity has been the single factor traditionally used to judge water quality and by this parameter alone we might view distilled water as superior. However, two other parameters need be considered when evaluating the "biological compatibility" of water. These parameters were established by noted European hydrologists, physicists and doctors in over 20 years of research. Important findings were made by the late Professor L. Vincent while serving as chief hydrologist in France. Based on his work, three parameters for biological compatibility were identified: Resistivity (purity), pH (acidity/alkalinity) and RH2 (oxidation/reduction). An instrument known as the Bioelectronic Vincent (BEV) was designed to test substances (blood, urine and saliva, as well as water) for biological compatibility. Ideal values were established and it was found by Vincent and his colleague, the late German doctor, Franz Morrell that only very few naturally occurring waters on the planet met the criteria for biological compatibility. They had originally believed that no treated water could meet these standards (pH 5.3-6.8 and RH2 between 25 and 29, as well as extremely high R). However, in 1984 Dr. Morrell endorsed the RO process as capable of meeting all three standards of biological compatibility.

While not all RO units meet these standards, the better ones do and the RO process itself would seem to produce a water of higher vitality than that produced through the distillation process which yields water which has often been described as "dead."

No discussion of water quality would be complete without mention of a major pollutant which permeates an alarming percentage of our water supply:

FLUORIDE

Sodium fluoride and sodium silico fluoride are by-products of the aluminum and fertilizer industries. In 1937 Dr. Gerald Fox of the Mellon Institute was the first to suggest that fluoride prevented tooth decay. Just coincidentally, the Mellon Institute is associated with the Aluminum Company of America (ALCOA). The sale of fluoride to cities for use in their water systems and to manufacturers of toothpaste, mouthwash, etc. presents a lucrative outlet for an otherwise useless, undesirable, *toxic waste*.

One of the most outspoken and fluent opponents of water fluoridation is Dr. John Yiamouyiannis (author of Fluoride The Aging Factor). Dr. Yiamouyiannis holds a Ph.D. in biochemistry and is former editor at Chemical Abstracts Service, the world's largest chemical information center. Serving in that position, he was in a position to gather much information re: fluoride. Dr. Yiamouyiannis opens his book by taking us to a village in Turkey where the residents age prematurely, exhibiting wrinkles and brittle bones, etc. in their 30s, with many not even living to age 50. Their condition is attributed to the 5.4 parts per million (ppm) of natural fluoride found in their drinking water. Where this same fluoride level is found in the water in parts of India, the same kind of age-accelerating effects are noted. (A certain amount of naturally occurring fluoride does not seem to produce such results, particularly when it is found in hard water which also contains high levels of calcium. Since calcium is the neutralizer for fluoride poisoning, fluorine brings its own antidote.) It is interesting, with this in mind, that one of the original studies supporting the use of sodium fluoride to reduce tooth decay was done in the town of Hereford, Texas in the 40s, where the townspeople's low incidence of dental caries was attributed to the relatively high content of natural fluorine in their water. This study was sponsored by guess who? - the Aluminum Trust! It was followed by a study in New York involving a large number of school children in two nearby communities, Kingston and Newburgh. It was reported, **by the Aluminum Trust**, that the Newburgh kids, drinking fluoridated water had 60% fewer cavities than their Kingston counterparts who drank unfluoridated water. Follow-up studies by objective sources have not upheld these results. The 5/89 edition of The

<u>American Journal of Public Health</u> reported findings by J.V. Kumar that the caries frequency rate was only **somewhat** lower in Newburgh (fluoridated) than in Kingston. It was also found that the decay rate has declined more in the **un**fluoridated city of Newburgh in the last 30+ years. It seems, as other evidence supports, that the use of fluoride only *delays* the formation of cavities. And, while tooth decay rates are now declining in fluoridated areas, they are likewise dropping at the same rate in unfluoridated areas.

Dr. Yiamouyiannis, along with the late Dr. Dean Burk, published epidemiological studies in the mid 70s showing that cancer rates in fluoridated areas were higher than in non-fluoridated ones. Based on these findings, Congress ordered a 10 year study by the National Toxicology Program of the EPA in 1977. By 1989 their research was completed, but not yet published, as it awaited a "peer review". Their unreleased report indicated that bone cancer and bone tumors occurred in laboratory test animals from fluoride. Proctor and Gamble performed a study with similar findings.

In 1986-87 the National Institute of Dental Research gathered data on nearly 40,000 school children from 84 geographical areas. Under the Freedom of Information Act Dr. Yiamouyiannis obtained their data, analyzed it and found no differences in the percentage of decay-free children in the fluoridated and non-fluoridated groups and no significant differences between decay rates of the two groups. As a result of Dr. Yiamouyiannis' analysis, the EPA has suspended its support of fluoridation (<u>Washington Times</u>, 5/1/89).

Sodium fluoride, added to drinking water, is entirely different from naturally occurring calcium fluoride found in oats, sunflower seeds, mackerel, raw milk, cheese, garlic, beet tops, green, leafy vegetables, almonds, sea water and hard water. Inorganic sodium fluoride is an instant poison. Fluoride is listed in the 24th edition of the <u>U.S. Dispensary</u> as a known poison used to kill weeds and rodents. So, it is rat poison with which we are treating our cities' water supplies in the name of preventing tooth decay on the authority of the aluminum interests....makes about as much sense as disposing of nuclear waste in our food supply!!

Fluorine is not a mineral. It is a non-metallic gaseous element much like chlorine. It is given off in waste gases from aluminum factories. It has been found that the herbivorous animals in the vicinity of these factories exhibit signs of fluorosis (fluoride poisoning) after eating vegetation which has absorbed the fluorine through the air. Fluorides are formed when the fluorine ion unites with metals.

The U.S. Pharmacopeia lists some of the side effects that can result from the daily ingestion of the amount of fluoride found in 1-2 pints of artificially fluoridated water:

> black tarry stools
> bloody vomit
> faintness
> nausea and vomiting
> shallow breathing
> stomach cramps or pain
> tremors
> unusual excitement
> unusual increase in saliva
> watery eyes
> weakness
> constipation
> loss of appetite
> pain and aching of bones
> skin rash
> sores in the mouth and on the lips
> stiffness
> weight loss
> white, brown or black discoloration of teeth

The discoloration of teeth is known as 'mottling' and is a common result of fluorosis.

Dr. Leo Spira, who conducted experiments with fluoride on rats for four years found that it interferes with the proper utilization of B vitamins, damages the thyroid gland and kidneys and causes the heart muscles to become flabby and degenerate.

Dr. Yiamouyiannis reports that fluoride interferes with enzyme activity by re-forming hydrogen bonds. It accelerates the breakdown of collagen (the major structural component of skin, ligaments, tendons, muscles, cartilage, bone and teeth). This can result in the mineralization of tissues that should not be mineralized and demineralization of tissues that should remain mineralized. Mineralization has a hardening effect and demineralization has a softening effect. So, soft teeth and bones can be the net result of excessive fluoride intake, regardless of any immediate dental benefits that may be claimed. Dr. Spira lists otosclerosis of the ears (deafness) and sclerosis of the arteries among the symptoms of fluorosis. These involve hardening (mineralization) of structures of the body that should be soft. Dr. Spira also lists bone cancer as a consequence of fluorosis. Dr. Dean Burk, former chief biochemist at the National Cancer Institute stated that "more than 50,000 Americans a year are dying of cancer caused by fluoridated drinking water" and adds that "any institution who supports fluoridation is guilty of mass murder". Dr. Yiamouyiannis states that fluoride interferes with the use of oxygen in the body - **it depresses the synthesis of ATP.** With depression of ATP production, we don't have fuel to run the electrical generators (sodium/potassium pump) in the body and the stage is set for development of degenerative disease.

The June, 1960 edition of <u>The Herald of Health</u> quoted the then Medical Director of Marin County, California as stating that "fluoride is toxic to a segment of the population, the older age group, in that it interferes with calcium metabolism. It causes osteoporosis in the older age group; it has been known to cause tetany-form convulsions". It stands to reason that fluoride ingestion can lead to osteoporosis, given the disruption of the collagen forming mechanism that it causes. And yet some medical doctors today are actually treating osteoporosis with fluoride!

Over twenty years ago, the California State Department of Agriculture outlawed the fluoridation of milk and ordered fluoride removed from fertilizers **because of its highly poisonous effect on plant life** - and yet we put it in our water!? European countries banned fluoride more than 20 years ago.

The amount of fluoride used in water fluoridation is 1 ppm. It is not possible, however, to maintain a fixed dosage and the mixture may deviate lower or higher. Even at 1 ppm, fluoride use has been linked with birth defects, Mongolism, heart and kidney diseases, allergies and cancer. Dr. Sheila Gibson from the University of Glasgow showed that fluoride, at levels comparable to those found in the blood of people living in fluoridated areas, decreased migration rate of human white blood cells. This is highly significant, for it means that the immune response is seriously depressed.

Fluoride in the water can cause dangerously high levels of aluminum to leach out of food containers and cookware. It is also highly injurious to both water mains and water supplies. Fluorides attack almost everything and eat through metal materials. Analysis of water mains in fluoridated cities have shown concentrations as high as 8000 ppm (Concord, Massachusetts, 1/29/59 as per Standard Laboratories). Some cities have eliminated fluoridation strictly on the basis of increased cost of repair of water mains. Fluoride has been outlawed in Germany, Italy, France and the Netherlands.

Chronic fluoride poisoning effects the section of the brain concerned with volition and the will to resist. Experiments on rats have shown marked deterioration in mental alertness, accompanied by a state of 'passive bewilderment'. Zookeepers and animal trainers use sodium fluoride on their animals to pacify them. Fighting bulls given 1 PPM became so docile they refused to charge. Does this tell us something about the political ramifications of water fluoridation??

As of the early 80s, 108 million Americans were drinking fluoridated water and 25% of households used fluoridated toothpaste or other fluoridated products. Today most certainly the majority of households use such products, for it is no longer possible to buy a major brand toothpaste that is unfluoridated. About 60% of the American population now drinks fluoridated water. It has become widespread practice to launch fluoride campaigns in public schools and routine dental check-ups invariably include fluoride treatments for children. On 1/29/79 A New York State Supreme Court jury awarded $750,000 to the parents of a three year old Brooklyn, New York boy who was administered a lethal dose of fluoride during a routine treatment at a New York City dental clinic (the hygienist neglected to tell him not to swallow the solution).

"Effects of Chronic Exposure to Low Level Pollutants in the Environment" (a report prepared by the Library of Congress' Congressional Research Service for the U.S. House Subcommittee on the Environment and the Atmosphere) lists fluoride (along with chlorines, asbestos, nickel and mercury) as a pollutant which is dangerous due to its adverse effect on the central nervous system and the increased risk of cancer, heart disease and genetic mutations it poses. According to chemistry indexes, sodium fluoride is more toxic than lead and only a little less toxic than arsenic.

We seriously recommend that you take a closer look at the fluoridation issue. Find out if your water supply is fluorinated or not. If so, a water purification unit, such as one recommended earlier in this chapter, will filter out the fluoride. Even if your water is not fluoridated, chances are better than good that it is polluted to a dangerous level whether it comes from the municipal plant or your own well, so a water filtration system has become a necessity for almost all planetary dwellers. We further recommend that purified water be consumed <u>exclusively</u>. Avoid drinking water in restaurants and from water fountains. Carry your own pure water with you.

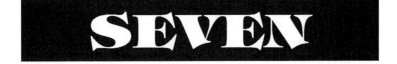

CALCIUM

We have chosen to discuss calcium to the exclusion of the other minerals primarily because of the 'calcium consciousness' the American public has developed in recent years and the misinformation that permeates that consciousness. Once again we have a case of the erroneous 'more is better' philosophy rearing its head. We have somehow allowed ourselves to be convinced through simplistic reasoning and the food industry's advertising campaigns that inadequate calcium consumption is a major cause of calcium deficiency and the consequent development of such degenerative diseases as osteoporosis. Believing this, conscientious 'health conscious' Americans are now increasing their intake of the popular calcium rich foods - namely dairy products. Our aim in this chapter is to address some of the popular misconceptions re: reasons for calcium deficiency and to identify desirable food sources of this important mineral.

Dr. Carey Reams believed calcium to be THE most important of all the minerals. He stated that plants, animals and humans need more of it by weight and volume than any other mineral. Dr. Reams observed that there are over 250,000 different kinds and 7 groups of calcium, one of which is toxic to all life. The body, he maintained, needs some of the other six every day. Calcium is the most abundant mineral in the body. Deficiency symptoms include:

nervous tension
tetany
bone malformation (rickets, osteomalacia)
osteoporosis
joint pain
muscle cramps and spasms
heart palpitation
slow pulse
tooth decay
insomnia
impaired growth
decreased glandular function
excessive irritability of nerves and muscles

No one would argue that the increased incidence of osteoporosis would be indicative of a widespread calcium deficiency. What is arguable, however, is the contention that this deficiency is due to inadequate intake of calcium rich foods. We maintain that it is not inadequate intake, but rather <u>decreased availability</u> of the mineral which is the prime cause of most deficiency conditions. We would also take issue with the notion that dairy products are the best source of calcium. The chart below (information from the U.S. Department of Agriculture and the Japan Nutritionist Association) gives the calcium content in various foods per 100 grams, expressed in milligrams:

DAIRY FOODS:

Cow's milk	118
Goat's milk	120
Cheese, various	250

VEGETABLES:

Turnip greens	130
Kale	179
Mustard greens	183
Parsley	200
Leaf-beet	100
Spinach	93-98
Watercress	90
Collard greens	203

BEANS AND BEAN PRODUCTS:

Kidney beans	130
Broad beans	100
Soybeans	130
Tofu (soybean curd)	128
Natto (fermented soybeans)	92-103

*SEAWEEDS(Sea Vegetables):

Kombu	800
Hijiki	1,400
Wakame	1,300
Arame	1,170
Agar-agar	400

*SEEDS AND NUTS:

Sesame seeds	1,160
Sunflower seeds	140
Sweet almonds	282
Brazil nuts	186
Hazel nuts	209

(* an average serving is 1/2 or less of the amount listed)

Also rich in calcium are many fish and seafoods, particularly sardines and shellfish. We do not recommend the ingestion of shellfish, however, for they filter bacteria, viruses and toxic substances out of polluted waters and concentrate them in their flesh. Please note that the seaweeds or sea vegetables, which are a mainstay in the macrobiotic approach to eating, are by far the richest source of calcium. These sea vegetables are also exceedingly rich in other minerals and for this reason are a helpful addition to the mineral poor SAD. Dulse and kelp are two sea vegetables that are not listed. They can be purchased in granulated form and make an excellent salt substitute. They're actually very low in sodium, but have a salty taste resulting from the abundance of other minerals. Kelp contains 1,093 mg. of calcium per 100 grams, dulse 567. The latter is the one seaweed that can be eaten directly out of the package without having to be soaked in water first. It makes a tasty mineral rich snack.

Notice that sesame seeds are very high in calcium. So too is tahini or sesame butter (like peanut butter, only made from sesame seeds). This nutritious food makes a good snack. It should not, however, be spread on bread, as this makes for a poor food combination (the protein of the seed + the starch of the bread). Try it on celery.

Notice too from the chart that the green, leafy vegetables are as rich or richer than milk in calcium. It is important that we consume these vegetables or their juices in their raw form so that we take in the calcium in its usable, organic form. Fresh raw vegetable juice is a rich source of readily available minerals, including calcium. Juicing is a practice which will eliminate the vegetable fiber, providing us with a rich source of vitamins and minerals in the juice. Juicing 1 lb. of vegetables is equivalent to eating 15 lbs. as far as nutritive value is concerned. A large glass of freshly squeezed juice has more food value than all three of the day's meals combined. When we eat a vegetable, 90% or more of its nutrients are eliminated in the fiber when it passes through the body. When we drink the juice of that same vegetable, however, we get 100% of the food value and we get it immediately, as the nutrients from fresh juices are available to the body in minutes. Hydraulic press juicers maintain more of the nutrients from the food than do the centrifugal force variety, but are more costly. A good centrifugal force juicer with pulp ejector can be very effective. No kitchen should be without a juicer of some sort. It is more important than your cooking utensils.

Getting back to the subject of calcium, we highly recommend a high intake of green, leafy vegetables (and their juices) as a superior source of calcium. Remember: The minerals (including calcium) from plants are organic and therefore can be fully utilized by the body. Once we have cooked the plant, however, or pasteurized its juice, we not only reduce the mineral content, but convert the remaining minerals to an inorganic form, which the body cannot assimilate and which will very likely end up as calcium deposits somewhere in the body and cause distress.

In support of the notion that it is decreased availability of calcium, not inadequate intake of it, that is the primary causative factor in deficiency of the mineral, we would like to cite some reasons for this poor assimilation:

(1) **INADEQUATE INTAKE OF VITAMIN D, MAGNESIUM, ESSENTIAL FATTY ACIDS (EFAs) AND SILICA**. In order for the body to utilize calcium, it must have sufficient quantity of vitamin D. This can be acquired either by ingestion or through exposure to the sun. The sun's ultraviolet rays activate a form of cholesterol in the skin, converting it to vitamin D. The type of vitamin D found in pasteurized milk is vitamin D2, calciferol, a synthetic form. In milk, this form of vitamin D binds with magnesium and carries it out of the body. Magnesium is essential to many body functions. The balance between it and calcium is especially important. If calcium consumption is increased, magnesium consumption must also be increased. The ideal ratio of calcium to magnesium is a matter of some contention. For years it was thought that we should consume twice as much calcium as magnesium and all mineral supplements were formulated using this ratio (most still are). In recent years, however, the efficacy of this ratio has been seriously questioned, by Dr. Guy Abraham, M.D., for one. He maintains (in issue #7 of Health Discoveries Newsletter) that the optimal calcium/magnesium ratio is just the opposite of what we've thought - 2 parts magnesium to 1 part calcium. He points out that man evolved on a diet high in magnesium (found primarily in fresh green vegetables, whole grains, seeds and nuts) and low in calcium. To increase calcium intake without increasing magnesium consumption (as we're doing today), he claims, results in premature aging through calcification of soft tissue. He points out that the body can store calcium, but not magnesium. Therefore, if too much calcium and too little magnesium are consumed, calcium deposits can build up in the body. Too much calcium in the cells will calcify the mitochondria, the power source of the cell and suppress ATP production, Dr. Abraham states.

Magnesium, he tells us, keeps calcium in solution and prevents formation of deposits in arteries and joints. The U.S. now has the highest RDA for calcium in the world. It was raised from 400 mg. daily to 800 mg. after World War II due to the influence of a medical doctor named Sherman who was appointed to set up the RDA for calcium. Dr. Abraham tells us *he had a big grant from the dairy council*. While the RDA for calcium went up, the RDA for magnesium <u>dropped</u> from 400 to 300 mg. with further drops anticipated. In 1989 the RDA for calcium for 18-24 year olds was raised to 1200 mg. So, our RDA for calcium is the highest in the world, while that for magnesium is the lowest. This being the case, if Dr. Abraham is correct about the ideal ratio of calcium to magnesium, we are creating more of a problem, rather than solving an existing one by adhering to government RDA standards and following the nutritional advice of the government. If you take mineral supplements, deciding on the correct calcium/magnesium ratio can create a dilemma under the circumstances. It might therefore be the better part of wisdom to look to food sources for these minerals, with an emphasis on fresh juices and land and sea vegetables. We can count on nature to know and provide the proper ratio.

EFA deficiencies can prevent assimilation of calcium, for these fatty acids combine with vitamin D to make calcium available to the tissues. We've already discussed the widespread deficiency of certain EFAs and the causes for it.

Lastly, the trace mineral, silica (found largely in plant fiber, most abundantly in horsetail and shavegrass herbs) appears to work with calcium to make strong bones. It has been found, in fact, that broken bones do not knit when there are high amounts of calcium but little or no silica. They heal well with an abundance of silica and the proper calcium in the diet. The French scientists tell us that the body can convert or transmute silica into calcium.

(2) **INTERFERENCE FROM CERTAIN DRUGS**. The ingestion of aluminum containing antacids causes an increase in calcium excretion from the body. TUMS is advertised as an excellent source of calcium. The type of calcium (carbonate) it provides, however, reduces stomach acid and since calcium cannot be assimilated without sufficient HCl, the calcium in the TUMS is not usable by the body. Corticosteroids (cortisone), diuretics and the anti-coagulant, heparin, also interfere with calcium absorption.

(3) **LACK OF EXERCISE**. Being confined to bed rest following an illness results in depletion of calcium from the bones and nitrogen from the muscle tissues. For this reason, physical activity is encouraged as soon as possible during recovery.

(4) **LACK OF HCl**. Most of us lack HCl due to overconsumption of protein, requiring an acid secretion for digestion. As previously mentioned, calcium cannot be assimilated in such an under-acid condition.

(5) **TOO MUCH DIETARY FAT**. Excess fat combines with calcium to form insoluble calcium soaps which cannot be assimilated.

(6) **TOO MUCH PHOSPHORUS**. A ratio of 2.5 parts calcium to 1 part phosphorus in the bones is maintained by the healthy body. Meat is very high in phosphorus. So are soft drinks which contain phosphoric acid (to keep the bubbles from going flat). Overconsumption of both of these creates an excess intake of phosphorus and throws off the calcium/phosphorus ratio. Phosphoric acid in sodas binds with magnesium and pulls both minerals out of the body.

(7) **FLUOROSIS**. Fluoride poisoning, as previously discussed, disrupts collagen formation, impairing calcium metabolism.

(8) **ELECTROMAGNETIC POLLUTION**. Dis-

cussed fully in chapter 11, we find that one adverse effect of high amplitude 'extremely low frequency' fields, such as found near high tension lines, is interference with calcium metabolism.

(9) **INORGANIC OXALIC ACID CONSUMPTION.** The green, leafy vegetables (spinach, Swiss chard, French sorrel, turnip and mustard greens, kale, collards) contain oxalic acid, which, in its organic state is beneficial to the body. It stimulates peristalsis. Oxalic acid combines with calcium in the body. If both are organic, we have a workable combination, with the oxalic acid assisting in the digesting of the calcium. However, when the oxalic acid has become inorganic as a result of cooking or processing of foods that contain it, then it forms an interlocking bond with any calcium ingested at the same meal and destroys the nutritive value of both. The net result is serious calcium deficiency. When oxalic acid is converted to an inorganic acid it often results in the creation of oxalic acid crystals in the kidneys. Calcium oxalate is a major component of kidney stones.

(10) **OVERCONSUMPTION OF PHYTIC ACID.** Phytic acid is an organic acid found in the outer husks of grains. When the whole grain is consumed, there is no risk of consuming too much phytic acid. However, when the bran and germ are removed from the grain and consumed separately in large amounts, we can have problems, for calcium tends to bind with the phytic acid and form an insoluble complex not usable by the body.

(11) **CONSUMPTION OF PASTEURIZED PRODUCTS.** The pasteurization process is discussed more fully later in this chapter. The point has already been made - and bears repeating - that the heat used in the pasteurization process converts organic into inorganic minerals which frequently cannot be assimilated completely. Calcium from pasteurized milk is therefore inorganic, and as such, is not fully assimilable by the body.

(12) **EXCESS USE OF ALCOHOL, TOBACCO, SUGAR.** Use of these stimulants increases the need for calcium to neutralize the acidity that they create in the system.

(13) **EXCESS PROTEIN CONSUMPTION.** Like the above mentioned items, over-consumption of protein creates an acid condition in the body, Calcium, being an alkaline mineral, is pulled from the body's own tissues to balance pH if a usable form of the mineral is not supplied in the diet. It is entirely possible to have the cells starved for calcium while heavy calcium deposits build up outside of them.

(14) **EXCESSIVE SALT INTAKE.** Table salt is an inorganic form of sodium. The more salt you take in, the more calcium you excrete.

(15) **OROTIC ACID DEFICIENCY.** Inability of the body to synthesize this element of the B complex will adversely affect calcium utilization, for orotic acid pulls calcium into the bones. If our livers aren't able to produce orotic acid, instead of getting into the bones, calcium is deposited in soft tissues.

It is not difficult to get calcium into the stomach and blood circulation, but it is not that easy to get to the cellular level, where we quite literally live or die.

We have already mentioned that the RDA went up to 800 mg. daily after World War II. For teenagers, it's even more - 1200 mg. daily. Many nutritionists recommend a daily intake of between 1000 and 1500 mg. Since the SAD typically contains only 450 - 500 mg. of calcium, it is tempting to conclude that we are not taking in enough. Dr. West tells us, however, that of 800 mg. of calcium consumed daily, 700 are excreted in the feces and that portion of the remaining 100 that is not stored in the bones is eventually excreted in the urine. The body's actual calcium requirements are very low, he concludes, maintaining that fruits, vegetables and whole grains can easily supply the needed amount.

He also points out, as we have mentioned, that excess calcium is picked up by the blood and deposited in soft tissues. He states additionally that excessive intake of calcium prevents phosphate absorption by forming insoluble phosphate products. This draining of phosphorus out of the body interferes with ATP production (and therefore the production of electrical energy).

Osteoporosis is a condition of too little bone mass. The bones in an osteoporosis victim are brittle, weak and very susceptible to fracture. Usually the disease is not diagnosed until a person falls down, breaks a bone and the x-ray reveals a bone mass that looks like Swiss cheese. Osteoporosis affects 15 million Americans and is present today in women as young as 25 years of age. Women need more calcium than do men and are eight times more likely to develop osteoporosis than men. Men are not exempt, however. We have all seen the stooped over little old man whose spine is crooked because the vertebrae have collapsed due to osteoporosis.

99% of the body's calcium is stored in the bones and teeth. The other 1% is in the blood for use in such vital functions as contraction of heart muscles, clotting of blood and beating of the heart. To maintain life, the body will see to it that a sufficient blood level of calcium is maintained and will steal from the bones and teeth, if necessary, to do so. For this reason, blood tests do not provide reliable measures of calcium levels in the body. The serum calcium level is not indicative of how much calcium there is in the cell system. We may have a normal level of calcium in the blood and still have bones that look like Swiss cheese.

Before 1970 osteoporosis could not be diagnosed until weakened bones broke and x-rays revealed reduced bone density. Now we have a means of diagnosing the disease through a process known as absorptiometry. It measures transmission of gamma rays through the skeleton using a small gamma ray source. This process has not come into general use, however, and so there is no commonly available means of diagnosing the disease. Even if there were, there is no cure for osteoporosis known to the medical profession. More than likely a medical doctor will advise the osteoporosis patient to eat dairy products and take calcium supplements, which will aggravate the condition, especially if the calcium supplement is of the inorganic variety. Pasteurized dairy products are undesirable for the osteoporosis patient, not alone because of the inorganic form of their calcium, but also because they are high in protein and are acid forming in the body. And the more acid forming foods we consume, the higher our need for alkaline mineral to buffer the acid. If we take in unusable forms of the mineral, not only will calcium deposits form, but the bones and teeth will ultimately be robbed to supply the needed alkaline substance.

If dairy products prevented osteoporosis, we should have a very low incidence of it, for we consume more dairy products than any other country in the world - 300 pounds per person per year! - and yet our incidence of the disease is very high. In fact, *the highest incidence of osteoporosis occurs in countries where dairy products and calcium supplements are consumed in the greatest quantity and the lowest incidence is in countries where the least amount of these products is consumed.*

MILK

As you may have gathered by now, we do not consider milk to be an acceptable source of calcium - at least not pasteurized, homogenized cow's milk. While raw milk provides us with a source of organic calcium, when the milk is heated to 115°C, the soluble calcium becomes insoluble so the body can't digest it. As Dr. Norman Walker observes, temperatures from 190° - 230° are required to kill such pathogenic organisms as typhoid, bacilli coli, tuberculosis and undulent fever. In the pasteurization process, however, temperatures between 145° and 170° are used. True: This process does kill some harmful bacteria, but it also destroys beneficial bacteria, whose job it is to keep the putrefactive bacteria in check. Ironically, then, pasteurization destroys the germicidal properties of milk. It also destroys vitamins, minerals and enzymes (including phosphatase, which is necessary for the assimilation of calcium). It changes the chemical structure of the protein and renders it and the minerals less digestible and assimilable. "Yes, but it kills bad germs", your conditioning may be asserting. Consider this: *within 24-48 hours after pasteurization, the amount of bacteria in the milk doubles!* We agree that it is of utmost importance that milk be produced and handled under sanitary conditions, but 'pasteurized' does not mean the same as 'clean'; it means heated. Pasteurized milk can be unclean and the process can actually serve to mask the spoilage. Pasteurization was initiated in 1895. As its use became more widespread, the health of the nation declined. Pasteurized, homogenized cow's milk is extremely mucous forming and very constipating. Even baby cows cannot tolerate it. Studies have shown that calves fed such milk died in 30 days! (Nature Has a Remedy by Dr. Bernard Jensen). It is interesting too that juvenile delinquency is highly correlated with high intake of pasteurized cow's milk.

So, what are the alternatives to drinking pasteurized, homogenized milk? There are two: Drink raw milk or don't drink milk. If you are over 4 years old, the latter is not a bad alternative. We are the only animal that continues to drink milk after we have been weaned. There are two elements in milk that have to be broken down - lactose and casein. The breakdown of lactose requires the presence of the enzyme, lactase, which is not present in 98% of the adult population, thus the prevalence of 'lactose intolerance'. Casein is the protein component in milk. Its breakdown requires the presence of the enzyme rennin which is gone in most of us by age 3 or 4. The casein content in cow's milk is **300 times higher than in mother's milk.** Casein is a tenacious adhesive glue used to glue wood together. Mucous production is a byproduct of the bacterial decomposition of casein in the body. So, there is ample reason to give up milk if you are an adult.

The other option is to use raw milk and raw milk products. In many states it is illegal to buy and sell raw milk. Some may legally deal in 'medically certified raw milk', milk which is certified to have been produced under sanitary conditions. Even in states where raw milk cannot be legally obtained, it is often possible to legally purchase raw milk products, such as cheese and butter through health food stores.

Apart from the issue of raw vs. pasteurized, we would like to consider the animals from which the milk comes. If you must drink the milk of another species, we recommend goat's milk as superior to cow's. It is easier to digest (20 minutes vs. 2-3 hours) and assimilate and it is closer in chemical composition to human milk than any other known milk. The baby goat weighs 6-10 lbs., about the same as a human infant. The newborn calf, on the other hand, is a tremendously large animal in comparison, weighing approximately 65 lbs. It is not surprising that the chemical composition of the milk of such an animal is vastly different than human milk. The fat globules in cow's milk are too large for the human body to process, while goat's milk is naturally homogenized. Drinking goat's milk might seem exotic to us, but actually 3/5 of the world's population drinks it. The goat is the healthiest domestic animal known and her milk contains more vitamins than any other food on the planet. Goat's milk is excellent for stomach conditions and kidney disturbances. Dr. Bernard Jensen (Nature Has a Remedy) recommends its use for babies and invalids in such conditions as tuberculosis, constipation, malnutrition, rickets, anemia, nervousness, weight loss, stomach ulcers and asthma. He emphasizes its germicidal effect and its ability to clear catarrhal conditions due to a high fluorin content. The benefits spoken of here apply only to RAW goat's milk. The pasteurized variety is to be avoided. While goat's milk is naturally homogenized, the homogenization of cow's milk is a process devised by man about which we have as much concern as pasteurization.

HOMOGENIZATION

Homogenizing milk changes the structure of its fat molecules. It breaks them up into tiny particles so that they are evenly distributed. Unhomogenized cow's milk has cream floating on the top.

Research by Dr. Kurt A. Oster, a leading cardiologist (as reported in the 8/78 issue of <u>Acres USA</u>) cited homogenized milk as a major cause of heart disease in this country. The following year, it was reported that Dr. Kurt Esselbacher, chairman of Harvard Medical School's Department of Medicine, drew the same conclusion: "homogenized milk, because of its XO content (an enzyme, xanthine oxidase), is one of the major causes of heart disease in the U.S." (<u>Dairy Goat Journal</u>, 5/79).

In unhomogenized milk, XO is digested in the stomach. In homogenized milk, fat globules encase the enzyme. It therefore passes through the stomach undigested and enters the bloodstream. It has an affinity for a compound found in the artery walls, and, should it become detached from its casing of fat there, it will, via a chemical reaction, cause an abrasion in that artery wall. *The body tries to repair this abrasion with cholesterol, calcium and other minerals.*

All dairy products, including skim milk and ice cream, are homogenized. The homogenization process does not improve the taste or nutritional value of milk. *All it does is prolong shelf life.*

TYPES OF CALCIUM

There are many different forms of calcium (and other minerals as well) and it can be mind boggling to walk into a store and note all the different types. Our aim in this section is to familiarize you with these different types and to clarify some misleading labeling practices. While we speak of calcium here, what is said will apply to other minerals as well. We are not advocating the use of calcium supplements by providing this information, but include it for the benefit of those who may choose to use such supplements.

We have mentioned chelation previously. You will recall that the word is derived from the Greek word 'chele' which means 'claw' and that chelated calcium is therefore bound (or held in a claw-like fashion) to another substance. It is that other substance which is known as the chelating agent and it determines how efficiently the calcium will be absorbed and utilized. There are two basic forms of calcium - inorganic mineral salts and organic chelates.

Inorganic forms of calcium are found in dolomite, bone meal and oyster shell. These include:

calcium sulfate
calcium phosphate
calcium carbonate

These forms of calcium are called inorganic because the calcium is bound to an inorganic salt: For example, calcium sulphate = calcium (mineral) + sulfate radical (inorganic salt). These inorganic forms of calcium are poorly utilized by the body, with an absorption rate of only about 5-10%. They are, as you might guess, the cheaper forms of calcium. Their use is not recommended.

Organic chelates are much more readily absorbed through the intestinal wall. They include:

calcium gluconate
calcium lactate
calcium citrate
calcium amino acid chelate
calcium orotate (no longer readily available)
calcium ascorbate
calcium aspartate

These forms of calcium are called organic chelates because the calcium is bound to an organic substance: For example, calcium gluconate = calcium (mineral) + gluconic acid (the organic chelating agent).

In nature, plants chelate inorganic minerals, converting them into organic ones. The human body, given sufficient HCl can also do some of its own chelating of inorganic minerals. Manufacturers of organic calcium chelates imitate nature in the creation of their supplements. They will start off with an inorganic calcium salt such as calcium phosphate (see #1, p. 145). The first step in the process is to separate the calcium from the phosphate molecule (#2, p. 145). A chelating agent (gluconic acid, for example, referred to as GA, #3) is then added. The gluconic acid, having a natural affinity to the calcium, forms a strong bond with it (#4). The phosphate molecule is then removed from the solution (#5) and we have calcium gluconate, a chelated form of calcium.

Organic chelated calcium is absorbed by the body. The percentage of absorption will depend upon the chelating agent used, as well as the person's individual biochemistry. Generally speaking, however, the following list gives an approximate idea of absorption rates:

calcium gluconate	25-30%
calcium lactate	30-35%
calcium citrate	30-35%
calcium amino acid chelate	65-80%
calcium ascorbate	85%
calcium aspartate	85%
calcium methionate	80-90%

Calcium orotate, offering an absorption rate up to 95%, has been removed from the market by FDA dictate. Pure orotic acid causes liver toxicity. The element becomes toxic in the acid environment of the stomach. Enteric coated orotates however prevent the release of orotic acid in the stomach and cause no problem.

THE CHELATION PROCESS

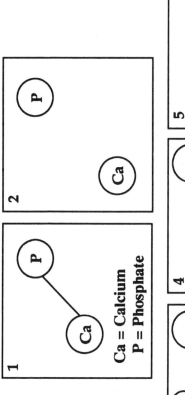
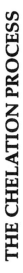
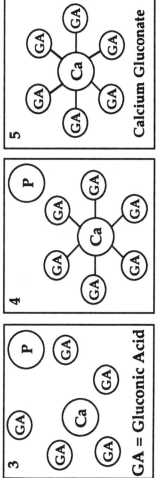

1

Ca = Calcium
P = Phosphate

2

3

GA = Gluconic Acid

4

5 Calcium Gluconate

Now, to reading labels: Can you tell the difference between the calcium content in the two labels below?:

1) Calcium (lactate)   1000 mg.
2) Calcium lactate   1000 mg.

It appears as if both of these contain 1000 mg. of calcium. In fact, only one of them does. That is #1. The word 'lactate' in parentheses indicates the source of the calcium. In this case 1000 mg. represents the actual amount of calcium (from lactate), also known as the amount of 'elemental calcium'. In example #2, we have 1000 mg. of calcium lactate (no parentheses). This means that the *combined weight* of the calcium and the lactate is 1000 mg. Since the bulk of this weight is from the lactate, the chelating agent, the amount of elemental calcium present is actually very small, under 100 mg. This kind of labeling can be deceiving. It is tricky, but not illegal. If, for any reason, you are seeking a mineral supplement, remember the information given and look for the amount of the elemental mineral, either stated as such or expressed with the use of parentheses.

In lieu of a store-bought supplement, you may wish to make your own. Try the following: Pour freshly squeezed lemon juice over clean, whole eggs in a wide-mouthed jar. Cover tightly and refrigerate for no more than 48 hours. Shake gently a few times daily. When bubbling stops, remove the eggs. Their shells will be soft, as their calcium has been leached into the lemon juice, but they can still be used. The lemon mixture you now have is pure calcium citrate. Shake it well and take no more than one teaspoon daily. Note that in this procedure no heat is applied. The calcium therefore is alive and usable by the body.

We hope at this point that the next time you hear the word 'calcium', you will think in green, leafy terms and not consider the cow. We highly recommend the complete exclusion of all pasteurized and homogenized dairy products from the diet. If you're a cheese-a-holic, consider the substitution of raw, goat's milk cheese and/or soy cheese (both available in health food stores).

EIGHT

THE WATER SOLUBLE VITAMINS

THE B VITAMIN COMPLEX

You may have noticed that we have referred previously to the vitamin B complex. It is now time for a formal introduction to this complex or family of vitamins:

> B1 (thiamine)
> B2 (riboflavin)
> B3 (niacin)
> B6 (pyridoxine)
> B12 (cyanocobalamin)
> Pantothenic acid (B5)
> PABA (para-aminobenzoic acid)
> choline
> inositol
> biotin
> folic acid

The above 11 elements of the B complex are official family members of the B complex, with the status of 'vitamins'. Those listed below might be considered step-children of the family, for though elements of the complex, they have not achieved the status of vitamins. For that reason you will not find them present in any multi-vitamin or B complex formulation produced in this country:

> B15 (pangamic acid)
> B13 (orotic acid)
> B17 (laetrile)

B13 or orotic acid had been widely and effectively used as a chelating agent prior to discontinuation at FDA mandate. Laetrile, you have no doubt heard, has been used as an alternative treatment for cancer outside of the U.S.

The complex of B vitamins works as a family, synergistically. The elements of the complex occur together in foods and therefore no one is deficient in any one B vitamin without being deficient to some degree in all of them. Because of their synergistic action, the taking of one or more increases the need for the others not supplied. It is therefore not a good idea to utilize supplements of single B vitamins in the absence of the complex as a whole. Even the complex as formulated, with the 11 vitamins, is incomplete in the sense that B13, 15 and 17 are missing. Once again, it begins to look a lot like food might just be our 'best medicine', for whole, natural foods are complete and balanced in their nutrient combinations and not subject to FDA regulations in their composition.

Generally speaking, the richest food sources of the B vitamins are liver, yeast, wheat germ and rice polish. The latter two are discarded in the milling process, so that the so-called 'refined' grains are deficient in B vitamins, even when they are 'enriched' by the addition of a few synthetic vitamins. Once milled, flour loses most of its nutritive value within 18 hours. In the production of flour all nutrients in the carbohydrate portion of the grain are destroyed. Furthermore, the chlorine dioxide used to bleach the flour is converted by the body to alloxin which has been found to destroy the insulin producing cells in the pancreas. Is it any wonder that the health of the American people has declined rapidly since the turn of the century with the introduction of pasteurization, homogenization, hydrogenation, chlorination, fluoridation and the milling process?!

Many of us have been taught that B12 occurs only in animal foods and therefore vegetarians risk developing a deficiency. According to John A. McDougall, M.D. (The McDougall Plan), however, B12 is only produced by micro-organisms such as algae and bacteria. The microbes found naturally in the mouth and intestines are the original source of the vitamin and, Dr. McDougall tells us, easily supply the daily needs of most people. If supplementation is needed, he and others recommend fermented soybean products and/or sea vegetables. Studies cited in the May '88 edition of East/West Journal, however, found that such B12 sources are unreliable. The article documents cases of B12 deficiency among some macrobiotic children. The question of whether or not strict vegetarians are getting sufficient B12 in their diet remains therefore a controversial one. It may well be with B12, as with so many other nutrients, that poor *absorption*, rather than inadequate intake is the problem. Dr. Rudolph Ballentine (Transition to Vegetarianism) points out that the less B12 we take in, the higher percentage we absorb.

B vitamins are meagerly supplied in the SAD, due largely to the refining of grains. The B vitamins are also depleted following a course of antibiotic therapy, for these drugs destroy beneficial intestinal flora that synthesize B vitamins. (These bacteria are best replaced with a rectal implant of lactobacillus bifidus or enteric coated capsule). Also, sleeping pills, insecticides, and estrogen create a condition in the digestive tract which can destroy B vitamins. A high sugar intake will likewise deplete the body of these necessary vitamins. B complex deficiencies are therefore very common in this country today.

The B vitamins play an active role in converting carbohydrates into glucose which the body needs to produce energy (glucose + oxygen = ATP). As previously mentioned, carbohydrate combustion cannot take place in the absence of B vitamins.

The complex of B vitamins also plays a vital role in the metabolism of fats and protein. These vitamins are essential for the health of the skin, hair, eyes, mouth and liver, as well as for the maintenance of muscle tone in the gastrointestinal tract.

One of the most critical functions of the B complex is its role in the normal functioning of the nervous system. The presence of B vitamins "may be the single most important factor for health of the nerves" (Nutrition Almanac, second edition, p.18). Three of the B vitamins - B6, pantothenic acid and niacin - play a particularly important role in reducing stress. Stress is anything that puts an extra load on the body - drugs, chemicals, infections, noise, surgery, fatigue, psychological upset. During the stress response all nutrients are needed in larger quantities, but the water soluble vitamins (B complex and C) are particularly subject to depletion, for the body does not store them. We have already established that B vitamin deficiencies are widespread. What happens then when the B vitamin depleted body comes under stress? It becomes ill. This has been established in animal studies. It was also established that animals were able to withstand the stress without falling ill when given a liver supplement, rich in B vitamins. Since the level of stress in our society is exceedingly high and the intake of B vitamins exceedingly low, we have a losing combination, a natural set-up for disease manifestation.

Though rich in B vitamins, the use of liver in the diet is not recommended. The liver filters toxins and, considering the chemical methods used to promote the growth of animals raised for commercial purposes, you can bet that their livers are quite toxic. Meat, including organ meat, is not recommended for human consumption for reasons cited in chapter 4.

B vitamin deficiencies can produce tiredness, irritability, nervousness, depression or even suicidal tendencies, as well as a host of physical symptoms. It is not surprising therefore that vitamin B complex supplementation has been effective in treating a number of ailments. Its use in the field of mental health has been

been particularly dramatic. Dr. Abram Hoffer of Saskatchewan, Canada was the first to discover that massive doses of B3 (in the form of niacinamide) could help persons suffering from schizophrenia. He gave psychotic patients 1000-3000 mg. at each meal and achieved a recovery rate of 75-85%. Dr. Hoffer has been successfully administering such megavitamin therapy for over 20 years. An entire branch of psychiatry - orthomolecular psychiatry - has developed using this supplemental approach.

One theory of why large doses of niacin are often effective in treating mental illness is that such patients have a higher than average need for this and other B vitamins not supplied in sufficient quantities in the SAD. For them, deficiencies result in more pronounced symptoms than for the average person.

The orthomolecular approach to psychiatry, we feel, is certainly an improvement over the traditional drug-oriented one. We do feel, however, that megadoses of nutrients, while useful in the short run to correct a deficiency state, are not a long term solution. Large doses of isolated nutrients can have drug-like effects in terms of reducing or eliminating symptoms and, as such, may be useful as an interim treatment modality. A cure, however, cannot be claimed until and unless the functioning of the body is brought up to an optimal level, with the normalization of circulation, assimilation, relaxation and elimination and the body's ability to regulate itself internally is restored. Getting the body to this point, we believe, requires considerable dietary refinement and lifestyle change. Vitamin supplementation can be highly stimulatory to the body if used in large doses over a long period of time. Increasingly large doses may be needed to keep us feeling good if the lifestyle changes needed to restore internal regulation have not been achieved. In other words, we feel that vitamin supplements may play a temporary role in the restoration of health, but that they should be a small part of the treatment plan and not the whole of it and that they should be used only for a limited period of time.

VITAMIN C

Vitamin C (the chemical, ascorbic acid, when isolated from its food source) helps build connective tissue by maintaining collagen, a protein needed for connective tissue formation in the skin, ligaments and bones. Collagen helps hold together all cells in the body. Because of its role in the facilitation of connective tissue formation in scars, vitamin C is helpful in healing wounds and burns. It also assists in forming red blood cells and preventing hemorrhaging and plays an important role in building immunity, for the white blood cells must be totally saturated with the vitamin to wage an effective war against antigens. Vitamin C increases the body's production and utilization of cortisone, as well as prolonging its effectiveness. Vitamin C, in conjunction with vitamin E and other anti-oxidants is required to block spontaneous oxidation reactions which create chemically reactive free radicals, identified as a causative factor in aging and degenerative disease development.

Vitamin C is found in most fresh fruits and vegetables. Some good natural sources are citrus fruits, guavas, ripe bell peppers and pimientos, the seed pods of wild roses (rose hips), tomato juice, cabbage and fresh strawberries. The RDA for vitamin C is set at 60 mg. (100 for smokers) which is a very minimal amount when we consider that an 8 oz. glass of orange juice contains 130 mg. of vitamin C. We must also consider the fact that the vitamin is water soluble and therefore not stored in the body. Most of it is out of the body in 3-4 hours. It is thus desirable to eat vitamin C rich foods throughout the day to keep the tissues saturated with this important nutrient.

Vitamin C, like the B vitamins, is needed in extra amounts under stressful conditions. Humans, unlike most animals, do not manufacture their own vitamin C and therefore must obtain it through the diet. Our vitamin C requirements increase dramatically when we're ill. Adelle Davis (Let's Eat Right to Keep Fit) tells us that 20-40 times more of the vitamin has to be given during illness to keep the tissues saturated. If we're undergoing drug treatment, it will not be possible to keep the tissues saturated with vitamin C, for every drug on the market destroys the vitamin and continues to do so for up to three weeks after it is taken. Smoking and the ingestion of sugar also destroy vitamin C. All of these things - drugs, smoking, sugar - are stresses on the body. In the stress response, the adrenal glands, which contain large concentrations of vitamin C, are taxed and the level of adrenal ascorbic acid is rapidly depleted. It is not difficult to see why many of us are deficient in this important vitamin. Many signs that are considered to be typical of old age - wrinkles, loss of elasticity of the skin, loss of teeth, brittleness of bones - are actually signs of scurvy, a vitamin C deficiency disease. Other signs of deficiency include shortness of breath, bleeding gums, impaired digestion, proneness to dental caries, swollen or painful joints, tendency to bruising, anemia, nosebleeds, lowered resistance to infection and slow healing of wounds and fractures. Breaks in the capillary walls are also signs of vitamin C deficiency. Since clots usually form at the point of the break, vitamin C deficiency can contribute to the onset of heart attacks and strokes.

A group of substances known as the bioflavinoids occur primarily in the pulp of citrus fruits. The bioflavinoids, together with vitamin C, guard the capillaries, prevent bleeding and provide a safe anticoagulant. These biologically active substances are especially concentrated in the white of the rind in citrus. They dilate the capillaries, increasing permeability, allowing absorption of more nutrients from the bloodstream. Vitamin C is 16 times more potent in combination with the bioflavinoids than it is when taken alone. For this reason, the vitamin C obtained from eating an orange will be more effectively utilized by the body than will the juice of the same orange, especially if the juice was extracted in a conventional citrus juicer. It has been found that there is ten times the concentration of bioflavinoids in the edible portion of the fruit as there is in the strained juice. To include the bioflavinoids in fresh squeezed citrus juice, it is advised that the fruit be peeled, leaving as much of the white rind intact as possible, and then sliced and run through a centrifugal force or hydraulic press type juicer.

The bioflavinoids are also known as vitamin P (think of 'P' for pulp). Some of their components are citrin, hesperidin, rutin, flavones and flavonals. They are found in fruits and vegetables as companions to vitamin C. *"They are essential for the proper absorption and use of vitamin C."* (The Nutrition Almanac). Think about that statement for a moment: The bioflavinoids are essential for the proper absorption and utilization of vitamin C. With this in mind, how much sense does it make to separate vitamin C from the bioflavinoids with which it naturally occurs? Proponents of the use of synthetic ascorbic acid argue that it is chemically identical to its natural counterpart. While this may be so, it does not contain the essential bioflavinoids. Once again, we are trying to isolate the 'active ingredient' and failing to acknowledge the synergistic workings of the natural elements, as well as creating an imbalance of elements in the body. It has already been mentioned that any truly all-natural vitamin C supplement (i.e., one obtained from food sources) would, of necessity, be very low potency, for a 500 mg. tablet of all-natural vitamin C would have to be the size of a golf ball. The higher potency vitamin C tablets may have some food sources in them, but they are primarily composed of synthetic ascorbic acid. While we acknowledge that the body's requirements for vitamin C are particularly high at times of stress, such as during an illness, and increased consumption of the nutrient is desirable at such times, we advise that natural sources of the vitamin be utilized and that concern for the quality of the source outweigh concern about the quantity of the vitamin ingested. Once again, the amount of the nutrient available to the tissues depends upon the amount *utilized* or *assimi-*

lated by the body, which may, and often does, fall short of the amount ingested. Remember: The bioflavinoids are essential for the proper *absorption* of vitamin C. During times of illness, therefore, it is certainly advisable to consume as many vitamin C rich foods as possible. It would be well, therefore, to totally exclude concentrated foods and take in only fresh fruits and vegetables and their juices. The old advice to 'get plenty of rest and drink lots of fluid' is certainly good advice; however, be sure that those fluids do not consist of pasteurized juices, milk, coffee, tea or tap water. Drink fresh juices. The key word is *fresh*. Increasing intake of fresh juices during illness will effectively increase the amount of usable vitamin C in the body, assuring saturation of the tissues.

For the above stated reasons, we make a distinction between natural vitamin C and synthetic ascorbic acid and recommend the exclusive, or at least predominant, use of the former.

Vitamin C has become a household word and once again the 'more is better' belief has been fostered, backed by supportive research. The research supporting vitamin C was funded by Holmes-LaRoche, the #1 producer of the vitamin. That research, we can be sure, was done with synthetic ascorbic acid. Vitamin C may be considered to be the 'active ingredient' in the natural vitamin C complex which includes the bioflavinoids. We've all heard of Dr. Linus Pauling, the man who made vitamin C a household word. Few of us are aware, however, that Dr. Pauling received a $1 million research grant from Holmes-LaRoche to study vitamin C! Few also are aware of the controversy between Dr. Pauling and his former colleague, Dr. Arthur Robinson re: experiments on the effects of large doses of vitamin C on rats. Dr. Robinson, former president of the Linus Pauling Institute of Science in Menlo Park, California, left the Pauling Institute in 1978 after 5 years of service there. Five years later, in 1983, Dr. Robinson was awarded $575,000 from Dr. Pauling as the net result of a legal battle between the two scientists. The details of this dispute are not widely available. There seems to be a great deal of interest - **vested** interest - in suppressing them.

A controversial experiment performed by Dr. Robinson is cited by him as the reason he was forced to resign from the Pauling Institute. Dr. Robinson reports (EIR, "The Nobel fakery of Linus Pauling", 8/28/84) that he had done research on mice which indicated that a "moderate" dose of ascorbic acid resulted in an increased incidence of cancer, while a diet of raw fruits and vegetables was very effective against cancer. According to Dr. Robinson:

The bottom line after three years of research was as follows: When you give mice the equivalent of the 5 or 10 grams a day of vitamin C that Pauling recommends for people, it about doubled the cancer rate. If you give them massive multiple vitamins, it does, too. As you go up in dose range, you near the lethal dose. And just under the lethal dose of vitamin C, there starts to be a suppression of cancer.

Dr. Robinson claims that Dr. Pauling suppressed this data which indicated that vitamin C was enhancing cancer at the lower doses and only suppressing it at the near lethal dose. He claims that Dr. Pauling destroyed his mice and 19 months later submitted a manuscript to him describing the experiment, *but* not mentioning that the lower vitamin C doses enhanced the cancer or that the doses which suppressed the cancer were *near lethal*. The paper, he said, submitted to him as a joint venture between himself, Pauling and others, concluded that if the dose were *doubled*, it would provide *complete protection against skin cancer in mice*. Dr. Robinson claimed that the double dose was lethal and none of the mice had lived. He therefore protested vigorously when this paper was submitted to the Proceedings of the National Academy and ultimately forced Pauling to withdraw it. Robinson claims, however, that Pauling later published it elsewhere as his own research.

Dr. Robinson is not opposed to the use of vitamin C,

but does express a concern re: the potential damage caused by high doses of the vitamin. Even the 'lower' doses referred to by him in his experiment are only low in comparison to the massive ones used, for his range was 5-200 grams (5,000-200,000 mg.). The following statement by Dr. Robinson (<u>The Healthview Special Report</u>, "The Great Vitamin C Debate", 1985) summarizes and justifies some of his major concerns:

Large doses of vitamin C have the potential to be very 'corrosive' on the body. When large doses of vitamin C react with oxygen in the body, dangerous 'breakdown' products are formed. These breakdown products are called peroxides and free radicals.

One of my former colleagues, Dr. Steve Richeimer, and I found that high doses of vitamin C will 'oxidize' into free radicals and peroxides and actually destroy protein molecules.

When Dr. Richeimer placed large protein molecules in physiological solutions of vitamin C, in a few hours there wasn't any protein left. It was just pieces. The peptide bonds of the protein were broken. Some of the side chains of the amino acids were also destroyed.

In addition, other chemical alterations in the protein occurred. Later we found this work was confirmed at an earlier time by Dr. C.W. Orr in 1967. Later confirmation was provided by the work of Dr. F.C. Westall.

Further review of the literature and chemistry showed that the nucleotide base rings of DNA are also destroyed by 'vitamin C breakdown products'. So now we are not only talking about the potential destruction of body protein, we are also talking about potential genetic damage.

There is still more. Dr. Stich at the University of British Columbia has shown that large doses of vitamin C can have a mutagenic effect on certain types of human cells. Mutagens cause cellular mutations and many of them will cause cancer.

As regards the potential destruction of body protein by vitamin C, Dr. Robinson suggests that this might be the reason the vitamin has anti-viral properties - it has the same effect on the protein coats of the viruses.

In addition to the concerns raised by Dr. Robinson, Dr.

Alan Goldhamer, D.C. ("Do You Really Need Vitamin Supplements?" Health Science, Nov./Dec., 1989) tells us that large doses of vitamin C can trigger a catalytic enzyme known as "vitamin C oxidase" which actually *destroys* vitamin C in the body. Then, when the large doses of the vitamin are discontinued, scurvy can develop as a result of the vitamin C oxidase continuing to destroy the body's vitamin C reserve. In addition to development of this rebound scurvy, ingestion of megadoses of C can produce diarrhea, raise uric acid levels and decrease urinary pH. This can lead to formation of urinary stones. Also, large doses of vitamin C can interfere with the body's ability to utilize other vitamins, especially B12.

Regarding the optimal daily intake of vitamin C, clearly the experts differ in opinion: Anywhere from the 60-80 mg. RDA to the 3,000-10,000 mg. recommended by Dr. Pauling since the 60s for healthy people. (He recommends 10,000-20,000 mg. daily for cancer patients). In between those extremes is the 250-500 mg. dosage recommended by Dr. Robinson and other authorities in the nutrition field. This amount can easily be obtained from the diet. It should be borne in mind that vitamin C is well absorbed at low doses, but with higher doses, absorption becomes considerably less efficient. Our stance on the supplementation of vitamins in general and vitamin C in particular has already been made clear, we believe.

NINE

FOOD SELECTION AND PREPARATION

Our intent in this chapter is to summarize much of what has been said in previous pages, presenting it in a sort of 'do' and 'don't' format. Some new information will be added as well, all aimed at giving practical advice that will assist the reader in making the transition to a more healthy lifestyle.

Before we begin our list of dos and don'ts, we'd like to say a word about where to shop. There are no blanket rules here. You may wish to turn to health food stores for some of your food items while purchasing others at the grocery store. A point we very strongly want to emphasize is that 'good' and 'bad' food can be found at both types of store. By 'good' we mean health promoting, while 'bad' infers the opposite. You must make your choices based upon an informed opinion. Between reading labels, visually inspecting food and handling it, you should have enough input, coupled with what you already know, to make intelligent selections. Once you are certain that you have selected the best quality food available, you will want to prepare it in such a way as to preserve its nutrient content. **When** to eat, **how** to eat and **what** to eat are all important considerations. We dealt with the latter in previous chapters and will summarize it here, as well as address the 'when' and 'how'.

FOOD SELECTION - WHAT TO EAT

- **Select fresh fruits and vegetables** - avoid canned and frozen.

- **Buy organic produce whenever possible.**

- **Look for a sweet taste in fruits and vegetables.**

- **Buy locally grown produce whenever possible.**

- **Eat food as soon after it is harvested as possible.**

- **Do not buy or use white sugar -** substitute molasses, stevia or maple syrup.

- **Avoid all refined and processed foods -** Select fresh, complete foods.

- **Do not buy or use table salt -** substitute dulse or kelp or a blend of herbs and spices.

- **Use only unrefined oils and oil products and use them sparingly.**

- **Avoid all hydrogenated oil products** (margarine, shortening, most commercial peanut butters, processed cheeses) and processed foods in which they're found.

- **Avoid all homogenized, pasteurized products.**

- **If you must eat cheese, choose raw goat cheese or soy cheese.**

- **Never buy orange cheeses.** ('Cheese Whiz' and 'Velveeta' don't even meet the federal definition of cheese.)

- **Beware of 'all natural' labels.**

- **Do not use black pepper** (it irritates the GI tract), try cayenne instead.

162

- **Use goat's milk instead of cow's milk and drink it raw.** If you can buy only pasteurized, drink something else!

- **Use leaf lettuce, Boston or Romaine** - iceberg slows digestion and is less nutritious.

- **Use only <u>whole</u> grains.**

- **Select sprouted grain bread in preference to that made with flour.**

- **Avoid ground meats, pork products and shellfish.**

- **Select oranges and grapes *with* seeds** - the seedless varieties are deficient in manganese.

- **Look for potatoes without sunken eyes** (which indicate manganese deficiency).

- **Weigh your fruit - the heavier it is, the higher the mineral content.**

- **Avoid thick-skinned citrus fruit** - the thin-skinned variety has more minerals.

- **Select 'fertile' eggs** (available at health food stores) from hens that run free. All eggs are mucous forming, however, and should be kept to a minimum.

- **Avoid all foods containing preservatives.**

- **Substitute carob for chocolate** - it tastes much the same, but comes from a fruit and is alkaline-forming.

- **Avoid synthetic nutrients from processed food and vitamin supplements.**

- **Read Labels.**

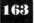

Avoid canned and bottled juices. Prepare fresh.

If you see it advertised, don't buy it!

FOOD PREPARATION - HOW TO EAT

Refrigerate all oils and oil products.

Avoid frying. It devitalizes food. Adding fats to food makes it more difficult to digest. Lightly saute'. Use a wok whenever possible. Cook with olive, peanut or sesame - the more heat-resistant oils. Fats do the greatest harm to the body when heated with starches - i.e., potato chips, donuts, popcorn popped in oil.

Never boil vegetables. Saute' or steam them. Use a stainless steel steaming basket. Steamed vegetables are done when you smell them. If you cook them too long, the nutrients escape into the air. Never lift the lid while steaming, as you will lose steam, heat and nutrients.

Avoid cooking in aluminum vessels. This toxic metal is leached from the cookware into the food when heat is applied. Use stainless steel or cast iron.

Gradually increase the amount of raw food in your diet as tolerated.

Cook at low temperatures to reduce nutrient destruction.

Increase alkaline-forming foods (fruits & vegetables) to 80% of diet.

Do not drink tap water. Drink only purified water.

Do not drink fluids with or after meals. They dilute digestive juices.

Do not drink beverages that are too hot or too

cold. It hampers digestive secretions and may crack the enamel of the teeth.

- **Eat slowly and chew well.** Chewing well not only aids digestion, but helps distribute cerebral-spinal fluid which transports minerals.

- **Always have a salad with meat** or with a meal of other concentrated foods to provide bulk to move these foods through the intestines.

- **Prepare foods with a calm and loving state of mind.** Thoughts are things and their energy penetrates and influences matter. Do not contaminate your food with negativity.

- **Avoid large meals.** It has been demonstrated repeatedly that over-eating reduces life expectancy, while systematic undereating correlates highly with longevity.

- *Slowly* **reduce intake of stimulatory foods**: protein, sugar, coffee, tea, colas, salt.

- **Eat green, leafy vegetables raw only because of their oxalic acid content.**

- **Get plenty of fiber in the diet, but get it from fruits, vegetables, and whole grains.** Avoid eating the bran and/or germ by itself. Do not increase fiber in the diet too rapidly - the body can't handle it until we build vitality.

- **Soak nuts and seeds in pure water overnight to release enzyme inhibitors.**

- **Eat only one concentrated food** (low water content food) per meal.

- **Scrub fruits and vegetables clean.** To remove poisonous surface sprays add 4 T. of salt and the juice of half a fresh lemon to a sinkful of water. This makes a weak HCl solution. Soak fruits and vegetables 5 to 10 minutes.

- **Avoid snacking** (see below).

- **Combine foods properly.** Remember the two big rules of food combining: eat fruits alone and do not combine proteins with starchy carbohydrates. Improperly combined foods putrify and ferment, creating acid-forming toxins and resulting in gas, indigestion and heartburn. Most foods spend a minimum of three hours in the stomach if properly combined. If not properly combined, they are there for 8 or more hours. Most of us therefore have our stomachs full all the time. And, since digestion requires more energy than any other bodily process, all of our energy is directed to the digestive process, with none to spare for healing. Among the benefits of proper food combining are that it:

  ... improves digestion
  ... conserves body energy
  ... increases nutrient availability
  ... maintains normal blood pH
  ... simplifies meal planning
  ... decreases acid forming toxins
  ... helps eliminate constipation, gas, diarrhea

- **Cultivate variety in your diet.** Do not eat the same thing day after day.

WHEN TO EAT

Timing is critically important in all activities in life. And so it is with food. 'When' we eat is as important as 'what' we eat and 'how' we eat. We are conditioned to gauge mealtime by the clock rather then by internal cues. Too often our eating is guided by habit rather than appetite and is done almost unconsciously with no real regard nor reverence for the food. In consideration of 'when' to eat:

- **Do not eat when under stress** even if it's time to eat, even if the food is on the table. Even the most nutritious food will poison the agitated body, for the meal will not be properly digested and assimilated and therefore will create acid forming toxins.

- **Avoid eating when fatigued**. Fatigue is a form of stress and the above applies to it. When we are tired, we need to rest, to sleep, and our sleep will not be restful if the body's energy is engaged in the digestive process at that time.

- **Do not eat unless hungry**. If you're hungry all the time, you probably have too much poison in your system.

- **Do not eat late at night** (see below).

- **Eat a light, simple breakfast**.

This last piece of advice may well be contrary to all the 'shoulds' you've ever heard. But actually, it's good common sense when we look at the amount of time it takes to digest what is typically considered a 'good' breakfast in the SAD: Bacon, eggs, toast, juice and coffee...**poor food combining**, resulting in foods being destined to spend 8+ hours in the stomach alone trying to be digested. And since energy can't even start to be *built* until the food moves into the intestines *and* since digestion is the body's biggest energy *drain*, it makes good sense that this big breakfast doesn't *give* us energy, *it takes it*!

We believe there is some merit in the Hygienist's recommendation that we eat 'fruit only' in the morning until noon (provided that the blood sugar is stable and that the body has reached a state of health and vitality where stimulants can be abandoned for this period of time without causing undue distress). Fruits are pre-digested. They do not require enzymatic digestion. Their proteins are already in the form of amino acids, their carbohydrates already in the form of simple sugars and their fats have been broken down already into fatty acids. Fruit therefore does not digest in the stomach and is only there for 20-30 minutes (except for bananas, dates and dried fruit which spend 45 minutes to an hour there). Fruits break down and release their nutrients in the intestines. This *conserves* energy which then can be re-directed for other activity, such as healing and cleansing of the body. Eating 'fruit only' for breakfast then gives us energy, for it is a food that is quickly digested. We want to suggest however that if the body is not in a condition where it can tolerate fruit, a breakfast of complex carbohydrates, such as cooked grains would be the better selection.

The rationale for eating a light breakfast and for not eating late at night comes from observation of the following body cycle:

8 PM - 4 AM **Assimilation**
4 AM - noon **Elimination**
noon - 8 PM **Appropriation**

The assimilation cycle is a time for the body to process what it ingested during the appropriation phase. Prolonging the appropriation cycle by late night snacking or eating the fashionably late dinner throws off our body's natural cycle. The same thing happens when we eat a big breakfast before noon, putting the heavy burden of digestion on the body when it is in its elimination phase. We can best assist the body's eliminations by withholding food or consuming food which will assist in the elimination process. Fruit is such a food because of its high water content and short digestion time.

Through proper food selection and preparation - as well as good timing - we can assist the body in its self-cleansing and healing activities.

There is no one diet that we advocate for everyone. Some of us may fare better on a predominantly cooked diet, while others can handle a predominantly raw one. As the body changes, and the level of vitality increases, so will our tolerance for certain foods. So, our diet ideally will 'change with the seasons', so to speak. Also, in consideration of biochemical individuality, what is good for one may be not so good for another. We must cultivate the ability to 'tune in' to our body to recognize its needs. Taking into consideration our metabolic type can be very useful. This information, established through hair analysis, can help pinpoint our individual nutrient needs.

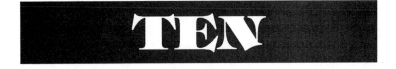

THE EFFECT OF LIGHT UPON HEALTH

There are two aspects of light with which we need concern ourselves: intensity and quality. Even the brightest artificial light is not nearly so intense as sunlight. In fact, it is ten times brighter *in the shade* than it is in the average artificially lighted indoor environment. Dr. Zane Kime, M.D. (Sunlight) tells us that this aspect of light affects our health, citing a rabbit study which showed that those animals, when kept in a fairly dim light, were susceptible to cancer, but that an increase in light resulted in a decrease in cancer.

It is the pineal gland, located in the center of the skull just above the eyes, that reacts to sunlight. This gland produces the hormone, melatonin, which helps regulate our internal clocks. The pineal gland seems to have a regulatory effect upon other glands as well and therefore its ability to initiate and shut off the production of melatonin is critical to the entire body.

It has been found that the majority of people over 40 in the U.S. have calcified or atrophied pineal glands. Such glands are no longer able to regulate melatonin secretion. A lack of melatonin production causes estrogen release. Overabundance of estrogen in the system is correlated with a high incidence of female type cancers. We find, however, that in the developing countries, where women have normally functioning pineal glands, there is a low incidence of breast and uterine cancers. Since it is *sunlight* that stimulates the pineal gland and the pineal that secretes the melatonin which has the regulatory effect upon the body, we can see that a lack of sunlight can actually be a *causative* factor in the development of female type cancers resulting in an overabundance of estrogen caused by insufficient melatonin secretion.

Dr. Kime cites Russian studies which demonstrated that laboratory animals developed "much less cancer" when given ultraviolet light (UV) by means of special sun lamps. This discovery was particularly interesting because it had been the researchers intent to *induce* cancer through the use of the UV lamps. They found, much to their surprise however, that it was not the animals living under the UV lights, but those under the fluorescent lights that developed the cancer!

It has become a popular belief that sunlight causes cancer. We maintain that, while overexposure to the ionizing UV rays of the sun can cause tissue damage via production of free radicals and consequent development of cancer or other degenerative disease, a certain amount of daily exposure to sunlight is not only harmless, but is in fact necessary for the maintenance of health. It was discovered over 80 years ago that sunlight has an important part to play in the functioning of the immune system. In fact, one physician won the Nobel Prize for showing how sunlight could heal tuberculosis. Other researchers demonstrated the sun's effectiveness in treating strep, staph and other viral infections.

The UV-C or far UV rays have bactericidal qualities. They are the most harmful of the UV rays and are absorbed by the ozone. The UV-B or mid UV rays also have the ability to kill bacteria and other micro-organisms. They play a role in calcium absorption as well. The UV-A or near UV rays induce the tanning response. This is the most healthful part of the UV and is necessary for photosynthesis.

When sunlight falls on the skin, the immune system is

stimulated to increase the number of white blood cells, specifically the lymphocytes. The lymphocytes produce gamma globin and interferon, immune serums which give protection from infection.

Because of its known bactericidal effect, sunlight was once widely used as a treatment for infectious disease. However, it fell into disuse when antibiotic therapy became popular. Today's medical students are no longer taught that sunlight stimulates the immune system. Instead, the harmful effects of overexposure to UV are stressed.

Apart from killing bacteria, sunlight has other known benefits. Sunbathing has been demonstrated to lower blood pressure and keep it lowered for up to 4 to 5 days after exposure to the sun. Sunlight on the skin greatly increases the amount of oxygen in the tissues and bloodstream. The oxygen, as we know, is needed in combination with glucose to produce ATP to fuel the electrical generators of the body. Lack of oxygen at the cellular level produces conditions conducive to impaired immunity and disease development. Sunlight also lowers blood sugar and cholesterol levels.

If all of this is so, if sunlight has so many *beneficial* qualities, why then is it getting so much bad press lately? Why has it become linked so strongly with cancer in the minds of most of us? Our belief is that under certain conditions, the sun can serve as a *catalyst* in the development of cancer, but under optimal conditions, its protective benefits are apparent. The 'optimal conditions' of which we speak are basically adherence to a healthy lifestyle and dietary patterns, coupled with a pollution-free environment. Such conditions are practically non-existent in our culture. But in certain more 'primitive' ones, where these conditions are met, cancer is unknown, despite heavy exposure to sunlight without the 'protection' of sunglasses and sunscreen!

The high incidence of cancer in our culture has, we

believe, a lot more to do with our lifestyle and environment than it has to do with the sun, whose rays are universally distributed and yet *apparently* nourish some while *seeming* to harm others. In looking at why sunlight *appears* to cause cancer, let us turn our attention to the subject of fats and what causes them to become rancid:

There are three conditions under which fats turn rancid: exposure to **heat, oxygen** and **light**. Our tissues provide the heat and oxygen. When we consume fat and then expose ourselves to sunlight, thus satisfying the third condition, we can be assured that the fat we have consumed will turn rancid (although chances are very good that it was already rancid, considering factors discussed in chapter 5, such as failure to refrigerate oils). Rancid oil, you may recall, gives rise to the development of free radicals, those renegade chemical fragments so heavily implicated in degenerative disease development. Ionizing radiation can also give rise to free radical production. Therefore, it has been assumed that cancer formation results from free radicals produced by the sun's UV rays. Could it be that it results more predominantly from the free radicals produced by rancid oil?

There are a group of nutrients known as 'anti-oxidants' which serve to **prevent** rancidity. These nutrients include vitamins A, C, E, the minerals selenium and zinc and the sulphur-containing amino acids. Many of these nutrients are **removed from food in the refining process**. Vitamins A and E, being fat soluble, are rendered unavailable to the system when mineral oil or hydrogenated fats are consumed (and mineral oil is a basic ingredient in many sun tan oils). Vitamin C, as a water soluble vitamin, is rapidly depleted under stress. For all of these reasons, the anti-oxidants are sparsely supplied in the SAD and therefore fats that we consume have little protection from rancidity. A study done at Baylor Medical College in Texas demonstrated that animals exposed to ten times the normal sunlight *did not develop cancer when they were given* *extra amounts of anti-oxidants.* The anti-oxidants then prevent cancer formation by guarding against rancidity. So, perhaps our society's proneness to cancer has more to do with dietary deficiency than with 'dangers' from the sun. It is plain to see how the sun can serve as a catalyst to accelerate rancidity of oils and fats, but the process **began** as a consequence of dietary inadequacy.

Anti-oxidant nutrients which guard against rancidity and subsequent free radical formation are found naturally and abundantly in whole foods. Once again, food processing is found to play a major role in disease causation due to the nutrient deficiencies that it produces. For the above reasons, a low fat, unrefined diet is highly recommended for protection from cancer, regardless of sun exposure.

The subject of light **quality** is addressed in the work of Dr. John Ott who has done extensive research on the effects of light on biological systems. His work and writings address the relationship between the colors of natural sunlight and our physical and mental health. Dr. Ott has experimented with what is now known as 'time-lapse' photography since he was in high school over 60 years ago. As a photobiologist, he developed the techniques which made it possible to observe the maturation of plants in minutes such as viewed in Walt Disney's nature films. In the process of doing this work, he found that, under certain conditions, flowers refused to bloom. In filming for one of Disney's episodes, he found that pumpkin seeds would not mature properly under fluorescent lights, but thrived if a UV light source was added.

Ott also found that light affected animal life in a variety of interesting ways. Fish, he found, stopped laying eggs when placed under 40 watt fluorescent tubes. When exposure to this light was reduced to eight hours, egg laying resumed, but the offspring produced under the pink fluorescents were all female! Reproduction normalized under full spectrum lighting conditions. 'Full spectrum' lighting is sunlight or an artificial light designed to approximate sunlight in terms of its wavelength composition. The graph below shows the wavelength or color distribution found in full spectrum lights:

SUNLIGHT

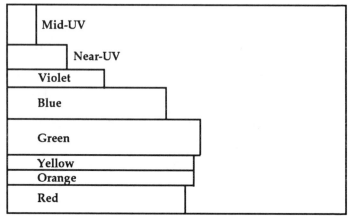

In contrast to the above profile, artificial lighting provides only a portion of the full spectrum. Note on the graphs below the unevenness of wavelengths in the incandescent and cool white fluorescent lights:

INCANDESCENT

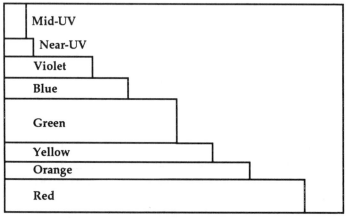

COOL WHITE FLUORESCENT

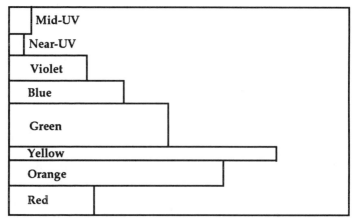

Notice especially the reduced amounts of near UV in the artificial lights. The incandescent light produces its maximum energy in infrared wavelengths, while the cool white fluorescent is disproportionately high in the yellow wavelength. Repeated exposure to such light produces a condition that Ott terms *malillumination'*. Light influences many physiological functions including our metabolic rate, respiration rate, blood pressure, liver, kidney and pancreas functions, immune response and maintenance of biological rhythms. Emotional stability is also affected. 2 - 3% of the middle-to-northern latitude population of the U.S. are affected by a condition known as 'Seasonal Affective Disorder'. This condition is characterized by severe depression and fatigue at the onset of winter and is related to diminished exposure to sunlight. Phototherapy (or light therapy) has proved effective in treatment of Seasonal Affective Disorder if it is sufficiently intense and is administered for a sufficient duration. The quality of the light is, as you might suppose, an important variable in determining the success of phototherapy. Studies conducted at the Department of Psychiatry at the University Hospital in Vancouver, Canada involving 11 patients during the winter of 1988-89 showed that UV light was more effective than both UV-blocked and dim conditions in treating Seasonal Affective Disorder.

Full spectrum light has also been used to treat psoriasis, neonatal jaundice, herpes simplex infections and skin inflammation. Light can help regulate the rhythms of the body. It has been shown to reduce high blood pressure, cholesterol levels and stimulate the immune system. Full spectrum light stimulates hormonal secretion and decreases work fatigue and eye strain which can result from artificial lighting conditions.

Prolonged exposure to fluorescent lights can cause a number of undesirable effects including eyestrain, headaches, insomnia, irritability, hyperactivity, fatigue and even increased dental caries. And yet these lights are routinely used in virtually all of our country's offices and institutions, including schools and hospitals. The British medical journal, The Lancet reported in 1982 on an Australian study which statistically linked skin cancer to a fluorescent light environment. Several follow-up studies supported these findings. Others did not, however, and the issue is not conclusively decided. None-the-less, Germany has legally banned the use of the cool-white fluorescent bulb in hospitals and other medical facilities.

Incandescent bulbs, as we previously mentioned, produce their maximum energy in the red end of the spectrum. Constant exposure to such distorted lighting can cause problems according to microscopic time-lapse studies of animal cells in tissue culture. In such studies, Dr. Ott found variations in growth patterns with different color filters. *A red filter consistently weakened and ruptured cell walls.* Ott also found that no mitosis (or cell division) occurred with three or more hours of exposure of cells to either red or blue light. Mitosis only took place under full spectrum (white) lighting conditions. Ott also found that he could increase the metabolic activity of cells or even kill them by changing lighting conditions.

Not only is the physical condition of an organism affected by light, but so too is the mental condition. Behaviors of laboratory animals will change greatly as lighting conditions are changed. Researchers have long known that it is necessary to remove the male rat from the cage before his pregnant mate gives birth in the laboratory setting, else he will cannibalize the newborn rats. However, it has been found that under full spectrum lighting conditions this does not occur. In a sunlit environment or one approximating it artificially with full spectrum bulbs, papa rat will actually nurture his offspring! To a lesser degree, humans seem to be similarly affected by light. Experiments carried out in 1986 in a classroom at Green Street Elementary School in Brattleboro, Vermont and reported in The Lancet 11/21/87 showed that children attending classes in the room illuminated by full spectrum lights took fewer days off from school due to illness than other students. In the 1970s, Dr. Ott set up a study in Sarasota, Florida where he resides. He introduced full spectrum lighting into a classroom at Gocio Elementary School and found that such lighting improved not only general attendance, but also the behavior of hyperactive children. Their learning ability and concentration were also enhanced.

In his research, John Ott found the key to the link between light and health. That key is in the act of light entering the eye. When light hits the retina, necessary glandular stimulation occurs. The pituitary, pineal and hypothalamus glands are activated. Light causes the pineal gland to temporarily suspend melatonin production. Lack of exposure to full spectrum light prevents the necessary suspension of melatonin production and can lead to glandular exhaustion. Under artificial lighting conditions, adequate glandular stimulation fails to take place largely due to the lack of the necessary UV portion of the spectrum. Glass has been found to screen out UV wavelengths. The glass found in household and automobile windows, eyeglasses and sunglasses blocks out this vital UV - and, far from 'protecting' us, can make us vulnerable to disease due to lack of glandular stimulation. Eyeglasses and contact lenses block 92% of incoming UV radiation. Sunglasses can be particularly harmful due to their tint which distorts the color spectrum. Recall the effects of blue and red filters upon cell growth and forego the rose-colored or other tinted glasses. Dr. Ott suggests that if sunglasses must be worn, a neutral grey color be selected, for it will at least cut down on all wavelengths equally. Special full spectrum lenses can be ordered if one has a need to constantly wear glasses. Otherwise, it is recommended that glasses be removed to allow the rays of the sun to act upon the retina, facilitating necessary glandular stimulation. To reap the benefit of sunlight entering the eyes, it is not necessary to situate oneself in bright light. The shade will do nicely. Remember: It's ten times brighter there than it is inside.

Dr. Ott tells an interesting story re: sunglasses in his book <u>Health and Light.</u> Engaged in conversation at a dinner party with Albert Schweitzer's daughter he was questioned as to the possible reasons why some members of a Congolese tribe had suddenly developed cancer when the disease had been previously unknown to the tribe. Speculating as to possible causes, he asked if houses with glass windows had recently been constructed. No. Had artificial lighting been introduced? No. Then, he half jokingly inquired as to whether the natives had been wearing sunglasses. Yes!! The glasses had been introduced into the tribe and were worn as a status symbol by the natives who frequently wore nothing but a loin cloth and the sunglasses!

Despite research supporting the beneficial effects of full spectrum lighting and the damaging effects of artificial light, the majority of our institutions continue to use the standard fluorescent bulbs. Why? For one thing we have - once again - the factor of vested interest. General Electric does not concede that light serves any but a visual function in humans. This huge and influential company does not recognize the effect of light on health, which Ott has devoted his life to proving. For a company like GE to adopt full spectrum lighting would be tantamount to admitting the inadequacies of the fluorescent and incandescent lights presently being used. Where then does one turn for full spectrum lights other than to the sun? In the late 1960s Duro-Test, which is the fourth largest lighting manufacturer in the country and the largest independent manufacturer began marketing a full spectrum fluorescent tube known as the 'Vita-Lite' under Ott's direction. It was this Vita-Lite that was used in the classroom studies in Florida. It was also used in a Boston study conducted at a home for the elderly. Here it was demonstrated that the rate of calcium absorption increases with the use of full spectrum lighting. While numerous favorable results were achieved with the use of this light, Dr. Ott was not satisfied with its performance, claiming that its cathodes gave off low level x-rays and that after about six months, the lights failed to give off UV radiation. He claimed that when he approached Duro-Test, they were not interested in correcting these problems. They maintain, however, that they did correct them. None-the-less, Ott went on to produce his own product, the 'Ott Light System'. It is actually an entire lighting fixture, rather than just a fluorescent tube. The Ott Light System, the Vita-Lite, and the Spectralite are presently the only true full spectrum lights on the market, for they are the only ones that produce a significant amount of UV light. To be full spectrum, lights must contain the UV or invisible part of the spectrum, as well as the visible part, for it is the lack of UV radiation in the commonly used artificial lights that seems to be the main cause of health problems associated with them. The Spectralite fluorescent tubes with patented cathode guards are available through Environmental Lighting Concepts (1-800-842-8848).

John Ott's work on the biological effects of light is now being carried on by Fred Mendelsohn, president of Environmental Lighting Concepts and Executive Director of Environmental Health and Light Research Institute, an organization founded by Ott which has done much to enhance public awareness re: the beneficial effects of full spectrum light.

Mendelsohn developed the phototherapy units used so effectively in treatment of Seasonal Affective Disorders. He developed these units in consultation with physicians at Johns Hopkins University. It was largely because of this work that Ott selected him to carry on his light research.

Mendelsohn informs us that both the spectralite and the vitalite are *ineffective when used in a regular fluorescent fixture,* for its diffuser prevents transmission of valuable UV radiation. Ott's light system is the only one that gives off full spectrum light and shields from the harmful effects of 'extremely low frequencies' (discussed in the next chapter).

Given the information presented in this chapter, the notion of protecting ourselves from the rays of the sun by wearing sunglasses that wrap half way around our heads and enveloping ourselves in a cocoon of rancid sun tan oil becomes ludicrous....

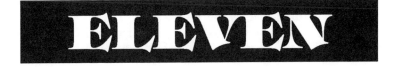

ELECTROMAGNETIC POLLUTION

Those of us who are old enough to remember will recall the controversy in the 60s regarding x-ray emissions from color television sets. Dr. John Ott, photobiologist whose work we spoke of in chapter 10 was among the first to identify this problem and attempt to correct it. He had read in the November 6, 1964 edition of Time magazine an article entitled "Those Tired Children". It described a case of 30 children all manifesting the same set of mysterious symptoms, all of whom had watched TV 27-50 hours per week. Symptoms subsided in those children who followed the doctor's advice of eliminating television viewing from their daily regimen. The article went on to speculate as to the reasons why the excessive television viewing would cause such symptoms as nervousness, continuous fatigue, headache, loss of sleep and vomiting. The speculation emphasized such psychological considerations as over-stimulation from program content. No consideration was given to radiation leakage from the sets - except by Ott as he read the article. He subsequently set up tests using bean plants and later rats to test his hypothesis and found that growth rate, behavior and reproduction were all adversely affected by prolonged TV exposure such as that described in the article. These effects were linked to x-ray radiation from the sets, for control groups exposed to sets whose picture tubes were lead shielded were not so affected. On the basis of his findings, Ott expressed the opinion that hyperactivity in children, which has become a widespread problem, may well be due to the exposure to radiation from TV sets. When Ott reported the results of his findings to two large television manufacturing companies, one did not respond and the other, RCA, conducted their own studies, finding their sets to be perfectly safe. Their director of research was quoted as saying: "It is utterly impossible for any TV set today to give off any harmful x-rays."

Soon thereafter, General Electric recalled thousands of their color sets due to x-ray emissions which they claimed were 'not enough to cause concern'. Later the U.S. Surgeon General's office announced that the issue of x-ray emission was an industry-wide problem and not confined to GE. Radiation levels as high as 1.6 *million* times the accepted safety level were measured by the National Committee on Radiation Protection. This led to the passage of the 1968 Radiation Control Act, setting limits on radiation emissions from TV sets. However, government standards were considered by many (including consumer advocate, Ralph Nader) to be too low to assure full protection. Since 1968, TV x-ray emission standards have been lowered eight times. And yet, it appears that x-ray radiation down to the zero level penetrates body tissues, causing subtle, but harmful effects. The closer to the TV set we sit, the greater the potential damage, and yet, at a distance of as much as 15 feet, reproduction was disturbed in Ott's rats.

X-rays are a form of ionizing radiation. When radiation strikes other material, it transfers its energy. At certain levels, it has enough energy to knock electrons out of atoms. This 'ionizing' effect breaks up the molecular structure and can blow the DNA molecule apart. X-rays, gamma rays (used in food irradiation) and some UV radiation are ionizing forms of radiation which give rise to the creation of free radicals that in turn are linked to symptoms associated with aging and degenerative disease.

The electromagnetic spectrum looks like this:

↑ COSMIC RAYS
  GAMMA RAYS
↑ X-RAYS
  ULTRAVIOLET
↑ VISIBLE LIGHT
  INFRARED
↑ MICROWAVES
  RADIO WAVES
↑ EXTREMELY LOW FREQUENCIES

Energy increases as we move from the bottom to the top of this spectrum. The higher the frequency, the shorter the waves. Below a certain UV level, radiation has a non-ionizing effect - i.e., it is too weak to rip electrons away from atoms, but at some frequencies it can still shake up matter and create heat, as is produced by microwaves, which are actually very short radio waves.

Radiation in the 'Extremely Low Frequency' (ELF) range is generally considered to be below 100 Hertz or cycles per second. Such low level magnetic fields were traditionally considered to have no effect upon bio- logical systems. Research has shown, however, that such effects do exist and can range from extremely beneficial to absolutely lethal, depending upon the frequency and other conditions. Our 60 cycle household current falls into the ELF range and un- fortunately this has been established to be a frequency that does not produce beneficial effects on living or- ganisms.

Dr. Robert O. Becker, M.D. did research with mice in the 70s to ascertain the effect of 60 cycle current. He exposed the animals for 30 days to a strength of this frequency that was equivalent to that found in the area near high voltage power lines and found that they demonstrated hormonal, weight and body chemistry changes similar to those exhibited by animals under chronic stress. By the third generation of mice there was a 50% infant mortality rate, as compared to less than 5% normal rate. The continuous stress response elicited from the experimental animals resulted in increased susceptibility to disease, for it exhausted the defense system. Dr. Becker concluded that in mice or in humans such stress could be expected to result in an increase in such conditions as hypertension and behavioral abnormalities, as well as an increase in degenerative diseases, especially those associated with decreased immune competency such as cancer. He also suggested that under such stress previously harmless organisms would begin to produce new maladies such as Legionnaire's Disease and Reye's Syndrome of that decade.

Since that time, the press has given much coverage to the controversial issue of the hazards of high tension lines and the overall effect of 60 cycle current on our health.

Epidemiological studies have shown higher-than-average rates of leukemia and brain cancer among electrical workers and among children residing near high-tension power lines. A University of Colorado study found that the death rate for certain cancers is twice the average for people living within 130 feet of high-voltage power lines. At distances between 100 feet and 2000 feet, the following have been observed: stunted growth, decreased calcium flow, abnormal EEGs, changes in blood chemistry and heart rate and drops in human reaction time. It has also been found that radiation in the ELF range can stimulate the release of stress hormones in chimpanzees, leading to immune suppression.

We live in a virtual sea of electromagnetic pollution with all manner of radiation being emitted from such sources as video display terminals, microwave ovens, hair dryers, electric blankets, beepers, water beds, standard household appliances, televisions, telephones, an array of sophisticated medical diagnostic equipment and more. To gauge the effects of 60 cycle current, hold a switched-on hairdryer in one hand and have someone muscle test the other arm (see page 31 for instructions). In all probability, the muscle will weaken, demonstrating the short circuit created in your body by the incompatible frequency.

Electric blankets and water beds can be especially harmful since we're exposed to their radiations for a prolonged period while sleeping. There has been found to be a higher incidence of miscarriages among women who use electric blankets than among women who do not. Miscarriage rates are also significantly higher (about doubled) among women who spend at least 20 hours per week in front of a video display terminal at their jobs.

Wall outlets leak radiation and if you have one at the head of your bed, whether turned on or not, 60 cycle current will be beamed at your head affecting pituitary and pineal function.

A Reader's Digest article ("The Menace of Electric Smog", January, 1980) tells us that, due to the electric (and now electronic) nature of our society, "the average American now gets a daily dose of electromagnetic radiation up to 200 million times more intense than what his ancestors took in from the sun, stars and other natural sources."

W. Ross Adey of the Brain Research Institute of UCLA did an experiment in 1973 where he exposed monkeys to the electrical radiation present in our every day environment. He found that the animals demonstrated changes in behavior and had a distorted sense of time. Adey concluded that exposure to electromagnetic pollution alters our natural biological rhythms. Artificial electromagnetic force fields created by power lines override the earth's natural magnetism and the body responds by adjusting to the pulse of the artificial signals, thus creating the stress response. The body's internal clock becomes altered due to decreased melatonin production by the pineal gland caused by ELF waves.

Soviet scientists have found that exposure to household appliances can cause central nervous system disorders. In vitro studies have shown that a one gauss field (such as found around household appliances) can significantly inhibit cell growth.

Russia seems to be ahead of the U.S. in their study of the effects of electromagnetic radiation. Their microwave emission standards are *1000 times* stricter than ours (their one *microwatt*per square centimeter vs. our one *milliwatt*. Much of our modern technology uses microwaves - radar, beepers, microwave ovens, CB and ham radios, remote phones and diathermy units). The thermal effect of high energy pulsed microwave energy is known to be damaging and was the only effect recognized by America when we set our emission standards. The Russians, however, identified a number of other effects including headaches, dizziness, eye pain, sleeplessness, irritability, anxiety, stomach pain, nervous tension, inability to concentrate, hair loss, in addition to an increased incidence of appendicitis, cataracts, reproductive problems and cancer. Non-thermal dangers have been documented in the U.S., but military and industrial spokesmen have refused to acknowledge them.

In 1959, John Heller found that garlic sprouts irradiated with low levels of microwaves showed chromosome damage. Also in that year, a Scarsdale, New York ophthalmologist began a study of the effect of microwave exposure on radar maintenance men for the Air Force. Examining the lens of the eye, he found no abnormalities, but, a few years later, he found that microwave workers tended to develop cataracts *behind* the lens. In 1964 a group of researchers at John Hopkins School of Medicine found a correlation between Downs Syndrome and parental exposure to radar.

One of the most dangerous applications of microwave technology was in the development of the microwave oven. When it was first sold, the maximum leakage permitted from the microwave oven was 5 milliwatts per square centimeter - five times the present emissions standards. Even at that, many recalls were necessary in order to fix ovens that leaked more than the standard. Research has not established that *any* level of radiation is safe. The effects of low level radiation are insidious because they cannot be felt and are cumulative. It has been established that the nervous system in humans is affected by microwave exposure which is 300 times below established 'safety' levels. In view of the evidence, we do not endorse the use of microwave ovens due to the fact that they all leak some amount of radiation. If you feel you must have one, then obtain a microwave leakage detector and check your oven at intervals.

In 1962 our CIA found that the Soviets were beaming radar-like microwaves into the American Embassy in Moscow. Although the intensity of the radiation was only .002 of the level considered dangerous by American guidelines, significant health impairments resulted. Blood tests of embassy personnel revealed that 1/3 had white blood cell counts almost 50% higher than normal, a sign of severe infection, also present in leukemia. A greater than chance number of appendectomies were performed on embassy personnel who resided on the sixth floor where the energy was the greatest. It seems that microwave energy attacks the hollow parts of the body (appendix, eyes, genitals) because reduced blood supply there makes these organs more susceptible to microwave thermal effects. The U.S. State Department did not take steps to shield the embassy from the microwave transmissions for another 14 years. As of 1980, two U.S. ambassadors present in Moscow at the time of the transmissions had died of cancer. The remaining personnel have exhibited a higher than average rate of cancer.

The Navy has experimented with ELF transmitters for 'communication purposes' resulting in the development of adverse symptoms in some of their technicians. Those symptoms included high levels of serum triglycerides, as well as a decline in the ability of some of the men to perform simple addition. For these reasons the Navy abandoned operating the ELF transmitters, we were told in a 1/80 issue of Reader's Digest. Dr. Andrija Puharich, M.D., LL.D. tells us otherwise. He speaks of other applications our military (and others) has made of ELF transmissions.

Dr. Puharich is a foremost authority on ELF. In addition to being a medical doctor and a lawyer, he is a physicist and inventor with over 75 patents in medical technology. He has also done extensive research in the field of ESP. Dr. Puharich claims that, beginning with Soviet transmissions on 7/4/76, many countries (including ours) have been engaged in ELF warfare, transmitting damaging frequencies to their enemies. These harmful ELF frequencies penetrate the body and influence cellular change at the DNA level, according to Dr. Puharich. They penetrate all barriers without losing their momentum, being stopped only by the DNA. Because it interacts with the DNA molecule, ELF can literally 'turn on' or 'turn off' any gene, once the correct frequency is known. Specific frequencies have specific effects: One can create a certain kind of cancer in rats in two days, another can reverse it. A specific frequency can turn off the insulin-producing mechanism in the pancreas. Depression, anxiety and even mob behavior can be induced by specific frequencies and this can be accomplished from the other side of the globe!

Dr. Puharich tells us that our military has conducted secret tests on ELF and has transmitted the frequencies, keeping the information classified. He claims that the CIA has attempted to prevent him from speaking out on the dangers of ELF. They have not been successful.

Dr. Robert O. Becker describes the first Soviet signal broadcast during the U.S. bicentennial celebration as lying between 3.26 and 17.54 megahertz - i.e., a pulsed modulation of a high frequency radio signal. This would place it technically above the ELF range. The signal became known as the "woodpecker" because of the tapping sounds it made. It was so strong originally that it interfered with several communications channels. Within a couple of years after woodpecker began transmitting, persistent physical complaints of mysterious symptoms began to be reported from people in several U.S. cities and Canada. The complaints seemed to be concentrated in Eugene, Oregon. The exact purpose of woodpecker is unknown. Becker, however, concludes that "the available evidence seems to suggest that the Russian woodpecker is a multipurpose radiation that combines a submarine link with an experimental attack on the American people. It may be intended to increase cancer rates, interfere with decision making ability, and/or sow confusion and irritation. It may be succeeding" (The Body Electric, p. 324).

In 5/90 the EPA released preliminary information about a draft report prepared by its Office of Health and Environmental Assessment which acknowledges a link between cancer and ELF fields. The director, William McFarland, stated, however, that the evidence showed only a *statistical* and not a *causal* link. What he did not reveal was that his own staff had recommended in the initial draft report that ELF fields be classified as **"probable human carcinogens"** and that this classification which would have mandated measures to protect the public health, was *deleted* from the executive summary of the EPA report after a meeting on 3/6/90 between agency officials and the White House Office of Policy Development (Paul Brodeur. "Annals of Radiation." New Yorker. July 9, 1990). The public therefore is on its own to uncover information found, but not revealed by the government.

It should be noted that not all ELF frequencies are harmful. Many of the physiological effects which are inhibited by one frequency can be enhanced by another. Certain diseases can be cured by altering the frequency (remember the work of Royal Rife described in chapter 2?) and the aging process of cells can actually be slowed down. Non-invasive genetic engineering can be accomplished through the manipulation of frequency.

Dan Carlson's application of high frequency sound to accelerate plant growth is an example of a creative and beneficial use of frequency. Carlson obtained the Guiness World Record for an indoor plant by growing a purple passion plant, normally 18" high, to a length of 600 feet! Application of his techniques has produced 20 foot corn stalks, 15 foot tomato plants, as well as huge potatoes, beans, collards, cabbages, etc. Carlson has developed a product which he calls 'Sonic Bloom' which he markets himself (Dan Carlson Scientific Enterprises, Inc., 708 - 119th Lane N.E., Blaine, MN 55434; 612-757-8274). The Sonic Bloom techniques consist of the use of a specific sound frequency around the 5 kilohertz range (identical to bird song) imbedded in Indian sitar music, followed by the application of a special nutrient solution to the plants. The frequency seems to open them up to maximum assimilation of the nutrients.

The most beneficial ELF frequencies, Dr. Puharich found, fall in the 7-9 Hertz range. 7.83 Hertz is the natural resonant frequency of our planet. This approximate 8 Hertz frequency therefore has a healing effect. So too does any harmonic (or multiple) of 8. This may mean that, had we built our electrical grid system on 64 cycles per second, rather than 60, we would be in a lot better shape than we now are! Dr. Puharich tells us the hands of the psychic or spiritual healer emit a constant 8 Hertz frequency.

Dr. Puharich's "Final Solution to the ELF problem" lies in the development of what is called a Teslar chip that he created in 1985 for the purpose of shielding individuals from electromagnetic pollution. This chip is housed in a watch and worn on the left wrist, for the left hand is the intake hand, through which energy enters the body. This device is marketed through ELF International, 1-800-245-0856. As public awareness grows regarding electromagnetic pollution, more and more 'shielding devices', which act as neutralizers against harmful frequencies, are appearing on the market. Other companies marketing shielding devices include:

Environmental Polarity Research
P.O. Box 22528
San Diego, CA 92122
619-455-5377

Energy Refractors
53166 St. Rt. 681
Reedsville, OH 45772
614-378-6155

Yao International
P.O. Box 0550
Murrieta, CA 92362
714-677-7869

An effective shielding device will increase the intensity of the wearer's aura and protect him from the ill effects of electromagnetic radiation. This can be demonstrated by repeating the muscle test with switched-on hair dryer in one hand, while carrying a shielding device in your left pocket or wearing it around the neck as a pendant. No weakening of the test muscle should occur. Such devices also help eliminate the effect of jet lag, which is a magnetic phenomenon.

Many companies have begun to market shields for video display terminal (VDT) screens. While acrylic and lead materials screen out UV and X-rays, they do not combat the microwave emissions emanating from VDT screens, nor the ELF and VLF emitted by the transformers. Televisions, as well as computers, radiate these frequencies.

In consideration of ELF warfare, as well as our use of 60 cycle current, microwave technology and all the other sources of electromagnetic radiation currently affecting our planet, some form of shielding device may well be an indispensable item of personal protection for informed individuals. It is also the better part of wisdom to avoid living near power lines and transmitting towers and to keep household appliances to a minimum (an electric toothbrush is not a necessity!). Additionally, it is advised to assure an adequate intake of the anti-oxidant nutrients (discussed in chapter 10) which provide protection against the effects of ionizing radiation. These are best obtained from whole foods.

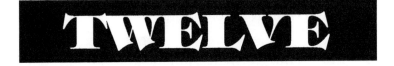

TOXIC METALS

Toxic or 'heavy' metals are minerals that are basically non-nutritive, that either do not belong in the body at all or are only needed in minute amounts. Largely as a consequence of the pollution created by our modern, industrialized society, these metals are finding their way in increasing quantities into our bodies. Heavy metal poisoning is an often unrecognized cause of many physical and psychological disorders. In the remaining pages we will identify some of the heavy metals and their sources and discuss some ways to prevent and deal with the problem.

ALUMINUM

By now I think most of us have gotten the word that it is not such a good idea to cook in aluminum vessels, for the heat serves as a catalyst, causing the metal to be leached out of the vessel and into the food. The same thing happens if we cook food in aluminum foil. It is probably advisable to even avoid wrapping food for storage in aluminum foil. Although no heat is applied in this instance, we believe that the direct and prolonged contact of the foil with the food *could* cause a problem.

Anti-perspirants are also sources of aluminum toxicity. In this instance, the aluminum makes its way into the body through the skin. Repeated use of these products can cause a toxic build up in the system. Read labels to determine the ingredients present in such products. A variety of non-toxic deodorants containing all natural ingredients are available in health food stores. Aluminum soda cans are another source of the metal.

Baking powders also are aluminum containing. An exception is the Rumford brand which has a cream of tartar base.

Finally, many antacids contain aluminum. Since Americans are now taking more antacids than any other type of medication, these products are viewed as a significant source of aluminum toxicity. We maintain that the high incidence of stomach and duodenal ulcers in our society is not due primarily to overacidity. Remember: Most of us are *deficient* in HCl. The putrefaction of protein may give the *appearance* of overacidity, but ulcer formation itself we view largely as a result of the inability of the stomach to produce sufficient quantity of protective secretions that serve to prevent the HCl from ulcerating surrounding tissue.

Aluminum deposits in the brain have been highly correlated with Alzheimer's Disease. Toxicity can cause gastrointestinal irritation and convulsions. Rickets can also develop, as aluminum adversely affects bone formation. Since calcium and magnesium are antagonistic to aluminum, adequate amounts of them in the diet will help reduce aluminum deposits.

ARSENIC

Arsenic is found in pesticides and insecticides and comes from metal smelting, coal burning and the manufacture of glass and mirrors. Toxic metals need not be ingested to do harm. Their fumes can be inhaled into the body and cause a good deal of damage.

Symptoms of arsenic toxicity include fatigue, loss of body hair, gastroenteritis, loss of the pain sensation and dark spots on the skin. Arsenic is a metabolic inhibitor and a cellular and enzyme poison. Trace amounts appear to be essential, however, for animals totally deprived of this element show a higher than average incidence of cardio-vascular disease.

High levels of this metal are rarely found in the body.

*LEAD

Lead is found in pencils, pesticides, fertilizers, some hair dyes and rinses, leaded gasoline, soft coal, cigarette smoke, cosmetics, pewter ware, and in some pottery which was painted with lead-based glazes. Such glazes sold in the U.S have warning labels cautioning the consumer not to use them on items which will come into contact with food or beverages. We cannot be certain however about the glazes used in either antique or imported pottery - these may well contain lead and therefore should not be used to prepare or serve food items.

Tap water is also a source of lead toxicity. It is estimated that one out of every five Americans served by public water systems consumes dangerous amounts of lead in their household water. Lead particles have even been found in the snow in the Arctic!

While lead-based paints have been discontinued, older buildings and items of furniture still exist which had been painted with such paints. Chips of lead-based paint, when consumed by infants or toddlers, can have devastating effects, for children absorb lead up to ten times more efficiently than do adults.

Polluted air contains lead. In the U.S. the average is in excess of 35 mg. per day, higher in some cities and in industrial areas. Lead is inhaled into the body, mainly from automobile exhaust.

This metal is a poison which blocks enzymes at the cellular level. It interferes with blood formation and is stored in the bones. Symptoms of lead toxicity include abdominal pain, constipation, fatigue, weakness, paleness. High levels of lead in the body have also been linked with behavioral disorders and learning disabilities. Alexander Schauss (<u>Diet, Crime and Delinquency</u>) points to studies reporting that lead levels found to affect the behavior of school children were below 1 mg., the level most commonly considered toxic. He also points to medical journal articles linking lead levels with hyperactivity, a problem that affects anywhere from 1 in 3 to 1 in 20 children in the U.S. Schauss suggests that the problem is so widespread that all correctional facilities should routinely screen their inmates for lead toxicity.

The following case history extracted from <u>Trace Elements, Hair Analysis and Nutrition</u> (Passwater and Cranton, 1983, p. 258) gives an idea of the potentially devastating effects of lead toxicity:

C.T., a thirty-three-year-old physician, became mentally ill with a diagnosis of paranoid schizophrenia. He was alcoholic and consuming large quantities of both drugs and alcohol while practicing medicine prior to entering a mental hospital. He responded poorly to treatment until a patient came to him asking for hair analysis. He had no prior knowledge of hair analysis and after looking into the matter ordered a hair analysis not only for his patient but for himself. He discovered very high levels of lead in his own hair, four times the upper limit of what is considered to be acceptable in our culture and also elevated levels of cadmium, mercury and copper. The lead concentration was by far the highest into the toxic range.....Following treatment.....his condition improved dramatically and his symptoms of mental illness reverted to normal....He lost his craving for alcohol and had no further need for psychoactive drugs.

<u>NICKEL</u>

Nickel is found in jewelry, cosmetics, cold waving (permanents) and in welded joints. Also, as mentioned in chapter 5, the metal is used as a catalyst in the hydrogenation of oils and finds its way into the body in this manner.

Excessive amounts of nickel in the body can cause asthma, skin problems, cancer of the lungs and nasal passages, brain blood vessel damage, gingivitis, stomatitis, headaches, dizziness, convulsions, back pain and sinus conditions.

Research has shown that "every second or third person has some kind of nickel poisoning", Hanna Kroeger tells us (<u>Old Time Remedies for Modern Ailments</u>, p. 43). She states that since opium is the antidote for nickel poisoning and poppyseeds contain tiny amounts of opium, taking one tablespoon of these seeds twice daily may help to relieve toxicity symptoms.

*CADMIUM

Cadmium is found in cigarette smoke, paints, contaminated drinking water, galvanized pipes, oxide rusts, welded joints and in shellfish found near industrial shores. It came to light in the press early in '88 that about 75% of U.S. seafood goes to market without being examined for impurities or tested for toxins. Expose's on filthy conditions in some seafood processing plants have caused closer scrutiny of the industry.

Cadmium affects the heart, brain, blood vessels, the renal cortex of the kidneys, as well as the appetite and olfactory centers. Toxicity can give rise to hypertension, kidney damage, decreased appetite and loss of smell.

*MERCURY

Mercury is found in cosmetics, fluorescent lights, thermometers, barometers, fungicides and hair dyes. Although not well known, it has been used widely in indoor paints to retard mold. Unfortunately its presence in paints was not required to be disclosed on the label. The EPA had considered regulating its use in paints in 1972, but was swayed against this action by representatives from the industry. None-the-less, in the mid 70s, DuPont, Glidden and Sherwin Williams voluntarily removed mercury from their paints. On 6/29/90, the EPA took more direct action and banned the use of mercury in all indoor latex paint. This action was prompted by the near-fatal poisoning of a 4-year old child in Michigan. This recent EPA ruling also requires that all exterior paints containing mercury be labeled.

Mercury is also found in fish from contaminated salt water and is used widely in dentistry as a major component of amalgams or dental "fillings." This is a source of mercury toxicity that we will explore more thoroughly since it affects so many of us.

AMALGAMS

In the 16th century mercury was widely used in medicine. It was found in ointment prescribed for treatment of syphilis. By the end of the 17th century, however, it was identified as a neurotoxicant. In 1685 mercury nitrate was used in France in the preparation of fur felt used in making hats. The workers inhaled the mercury vapors which affected their neurological systems - and that is the origin of the saying, "mad as a hatter"! Mercury has an affinity for the brain.

The first metallic fillings appeared in the U.S. about 1820. Six years later a silver paste which was a combination of silver and mercury was introduced. The silver came from smelted coins and so contained other metals as well; hence the name 'amalgam'. Previous to this time the only filling material used had been gold which few could afford.

The forerunner to the American Dental Association (ADA) was the American Society of Dental Surgeons. They stood in firm opposition to the use of mercury in dentistry because of its known toxic effects. However, in 1833 two brothers by the name of Crawcour set up practice in New York and exploited the use of amalgams by a rigorous and successful advertising campaign. They did a booming business, despite the fact that they had no formal training in dentistry. They were successful in creating a demand for the new filling material and attracted many patients previously associated with established legitimate dentists. This caused the dental profession and their society to retaliate, attacking the use of amalgams even more vigorously and eventually succeeding in forcing the Crawcours out of business.

For the next 25 years the official stand of organized dentistry was solid opposition to the use of amalgam. There were some dissenting members, however, and in 1855, to end the conflicts within the Society, most of the resolutions that prohibited the use of amalgams were withdrawn. The internal conflict soon broke up the organization. Shortly thereafter it was replaced by the ADA which has always stood in favor of the use of dental amalgams.

New amalgam formulations were subsequently developed and by 1870 the first organized movement in support of amalgams was launched. Claims were made that the material did not pose a health hazard. In 1900 Dr. G.V. Black succeeded in 'perfecting' the dental amalgam. Soon thereafter, opposition to dental amalgams was rekindled, due largely to the work of Dr. Alfred Stock, a German chemistry professor. In an article written in 1926 he identified dental amalgam as a source of mercury vapor emissions which caused the following symptoms: tiredness, depression, irritability, vertigo, poor memory, mouth inflammations, diarrhea, loss of appetite and chronic catarrhs. In 1939 Dr. Stock found the amalgam to be "an unstable alloy that continuously gave off mercury in the form of gas ions and abraded particles" (Silver Dental Fillings - The Toxic Time Bomb, Sam Ziff, p. 11).

It can be demonstrated by use of special equipment (the Jerome Mercury Vapor Analyzer) that the amount of mercury vapor being released from silver amalgams after the patient has chewed gum for ten minutes is excessive, often higher than mercury levels to which at-risk industrial workers are exposed. The implication here is that every time we chew (as in three meals per day), we are poisoning ourselves with mercury vapors, breathing in the fumes, as did the 'mad hatters' of 17th century France. This is quite apart from any mercury particles that may be leached into the system from the teeth themselves.

Today amalgams are 50% mercury. The other 50% is

a combination of silver, tin, copper and zinc. These dissimilar metals, placed in a solution of saliva, create conditions in the mouth conducive to the creation of electrical currents, for the saliva provides the needed electrolyte. The mouth therefore becomes a mini generating plant. In some instances people with enough dissimilar metal in their mouth can even pick up radio stations! This 'oral galvanism' initiates a breakdown or corrosion of the amalgam fillings, increasing both the amount of mercury vapor and abraded particles that can be released in the mouth.

The ADA in July '84 conceded that mercury *is* released from dental amalgams, but claimed that the amount released is too small to cause health problems, *except in rare allergic individuals.* This remains their official position. In formulating this position, Sam Ziff and Dr. Michael Ziff tell us that the ADA seems to have 'overlooked' studies which "demonstrate irrefutably that the percentage of allergy to amalgam and/or mercury can be as high as 44.3%" (The Hazards of Silver/Mercury Dental Fillings, p. 15). They also tell us (p. 16 & 18):

In the more than 125 years that the ADA has been in existence, it has not funded one single research project proving the bio-compatibility or safety of dental amalgams in humans....There is conclusive scientific evidence showing a direct correlation between the numbers and surfaces of amalgam fillings and the mercury content of brain tissue....Scientific research has demonstrated that mercury, even in small amounts, can damage the brain, heart, lungs, liver, kidneys, thyroid gland, pituitary gland, adrenal glands, blood cells, enzymes, hormones and suppresses the body's immune system. In addition, mercury has been shown to pass the placental membrane in pregnant women and cause permanent damage to the brain of a developing baby.

Dr. David G. Williams (Alternatives, Vol. 3, No. 19) tells us that "While interior paints were limited to 300 ppm and exterior ones to 2,000 ppm, maximum limits for dental fillings have never been set {and} silver amalgam fillings contain 500,000 ppm of mercury!

Dentists, with their constant exposure to mercury

have a higher rate of suicide than any other occupation (remember the mad hatters?). It is also interesting that cadavers of dentists showed *800 times* more mercury than those of non-dentists (Maine Times, 4/28/89).

There was a time when gold fillings were the only alternative to amalgams. That time has passed. Gold is still available, but new ceramic materials have been developed which are not only cheaper, but may be preferable. Although gold is relatively bio-compatible, the type used most often in dentistry is an alloy, mixed usually with palladium, copper or cobalt. The actual percentage of gold can vary from 2-92%

The newer tooth-colored materials are referred to variously as 'bonded resin ceramics', 'composite resins' or just 'composites'. These materials are demonstrated to have a high degree of bio-compatibility when placed properly. They are too new for any long term studies on durability to have been performed; however, "several 2 to 5 year studies indicate wear characteristics that are as good, if not better than amalgam" (The Hazards of Silver/Mercury Dental Fillings, Ziff and Ziff, p. 28).

You are not likely to be fortunate enough to find a dentist who will actually recommend replacing your amalgams with ceramic material, due to the ADA's official stand on the subject. For that same reason insurance will not cover the cost of replacement unless you somehow manage to demonstrate that you are one of the 'rare' allergic individuals.

Amalgam is also used as filling material in root canals. Dr. Weston Price, a former Director of Research for the American Dental Association, spent 35 years researching the link between root canal filled teeth and heart, kidney and uterine disease, as well as disorders of the nervous and endocrine systems. He demonstrated that damage to these organs results from seepage of toxins from the root canal filled teeth.

It is a significant development that more than 35 members of the ADA filed suit against it in 9/90 charging fraudulent misrepresentation and breach of contract (Chemical and Engineering News, September 24, 1990). This class action suit was filed in a federal court in Cleveland and charges the ADA with purposefully disseminating misinformation to its members regarding water fluoridation and dental amalgams for the purpose of protecting its reputation. This suit seeks monetary damages and an injunction which would prevent the ADA from continued dissemination of misinformation.

If you would like more information on this subject and/or the names of dentists who practice mercury-free dentistry in your area, please contact The Foundation for Toxic Free Dentistry, P.O. Box 580160, Orlando, FL 32858-0160 or call the Environmental Dental Association at 1-800-388-8124.

Mercury can cause cell destruction, block transport of sugars and increase permeability of potassium. Toxicity symptoms can include, in addition to those already mentioned, emotional disturbances, blood changes, chewing and swallowing difficulties, loss of pain sensation and convulsions.

DIAGNOSING AND TREATING METAL TOXICITY

Heavy metal toxicity often goes unrecognized and untreated, largely because symptoms are not correctly identified by medical doctors. The hair analysis mentioned earlier in our discussion of lead poisoning is not generally known to, nor used by, M.D.s It is more likely to be employed by a non-medical physician, a D.C. or an N.D. We do not feel that all such tests** will necessarily give an accurate indication of the amount of nutritive macrominerals present in the cell system, but they do accurately reflect the presence and concentrations of toxic metals. A small sample of untreated hair usually taken from the nape of the neck is used. Excessive levels of the heavy metals in the body can be reduced through either oral or intravenous chelation therapy or through the use of homeopathic preparations.

It is beyond the scope of this book to describe the practice of homeopathy. Suffice it to say that it is one of the oldest of the healing arts and is practiced widely outside of the U.S. It involves the use of highly diluted natural medicines and works on the principle or law of similars (like attracts like). Its effectiveness is not in the action of its physical substance, for there is little to none present in the remedies, but rather in the affinity of *frequency* that it has for the condition being treated. The vibration of mercury introduced into the body homeopathicly will, for example, pull mercury out of the tissues.

A chelating agent, as previously mentioned, is a substance which binds with a mineral, facilitating its transport either into or out of the body. Chelated minerals are bound with the chelating agent, usually an amino acid, which helps carry them into the cell system. Chelation therapy involves utilizing the same principle to *remove* toxic metals from the body.

Intravenous chelation therapy serves as sort of a chemical 'rotorooter' to clean out clogged arteries. It is a process that has been used in the treatment of heavy metal poisoning in the U.S. since 1948 and for hardening of the arteries since 1952. EDTA (ethylene diamine tetraacetic acid), a protein-like substance, is the most commonly used chemical chelating agent. Other potentially toxic chemical chelating agents include penicillamine and acetylcysteine. Specific nutrients, notably vitamin C and the sulphur containing amino acids, also have the capacity to serve as chelating agents, either directly chelating the toxic metals or supporting the body in its own efforts to remove the poisonous metals. Oral chelation is possible with the use of such nutrients, either in whole food or extracted form. Studies have shown that algae has effectively stimulated the excretion of heavy metals, including cadmium, lead and mercury without the detrimental effects associated with conventional chelation therapy.

We recommend the use of Light Force Spirulina developed by Dr. Christopher Hills. This algae is an exceptionally rich source of highly usable protein, as well as beta carotene (pro vitamin A) whose antioxidant properties guard against free radical production associated with degenerative disease. The decision of whether to use chemical chelating agents, nutritional supplements or natural foods will depend upon the severity of the toxicity and the judgment of the physician. If the physician is trained in homeopathy, that gives him a fourth option.

Intravenous chelation therapy is costly and involves repeated sessions of IV infusion. Treatments are generally given in segments of 12 and a total of 30-50 sessions are typically needed. The procedure is used not only in the treatment of heavy metal poisoning and atherosclerosis, but also in stroke, kidney stones, arthritis and bursitis and a number of eye diseases. Intravenous chelation therapy is not widely accepted nor practiced in medical circles, for it is a controversial alternative treatment. We believe it is certainly a viable alternative to coronary by-pass surgery! Please bear in mind that the purpose of chelation therapy is to remove inorganic mineral deposits from the body. These can be removed, only to be re-deposited, if the physician and his patient are not aware of dietary and lifestyle patterns that cause a build up of such minerals.

We feel that screening for heavy metal toxicity should be a routine part of any annual check-up, given the prevalence of these pollutants in our society and the likelihood of their finding their way into our bodies.

There is much we can do to avoid heavy metal poisoning and/or to alleviate the body's burden of inorganic minerals. We recommend going over to a pure water source (one devoid of minerals), eating whole, unprocessed foods, having amalgam fillings replaced with composites and avoiding the ingestion of inorganic minerals in supplement form. Foods which are rich in the sulphur-containing amino acids include beans, eggs, onions and garlic. Increased intake of these foods can help the body in its chelation efforts. Another natural chelating agent is algin, found abundantly in kelp. In addition, we can familiarize ourselves with the sources of heavy metal toxicity and avoid or minimize exposure to such contaminants.

---

* There has been no nutritive need established for these metals.

** Different measurement systems and norms are used by different hair analysis labs. One reliable lab is that founded by Dr. Paul Eck:

      Analytical Research Labs, Inc.
      8650 N. 22nd Ave. Phoenix, AZ 85021
      602-995-1580

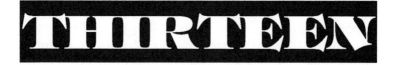

IMMUNIZATIONS

The word 'immunization' is actually misleading, for to 'immunize' is "to render immune" or resistant to disease. To vaccinate is to inoculate with a vaccine for the purpose of producing immunity against disease. To inoculate is "to introduce the virus of a disease or other antigenic material into the body in order to immunize, cure or experiment" (The Concise American Heritage Dictionary). We often use the word 'immunize' interchangeably with 'vaccinate' or 'inoculate', implying our acceptance of the belief that vaccinations or inoculations confer immunity against disease upon the recipient. This commonly held belief may be unfounded and invalid, as we hope to illustrate in the remaining pages of this chapter. Therefore, we will henceforth refer to 'immunizations' as vaccinations and ask that you consider doing likewise.

While there are no national vaccination laws in the U.S., there is a high degree of uniformity among the states on vaccination policy. All 50 states require vaccination against traditional childhood diseases as a pre-requisite to public school admission. The vaccinations required in all states include diphtheria, measles, rubella and polio. Arizona and Montana require only these four. Most other states require, in addition, vaccination against tetanus, mumps and pertussis. Let's take a brief look at each of these diseases and the vaccines administered to prevent them:

MEASLES

The live measles vaccine was introduced in 1963. It is
typically administered as part of the MMR (Measles,
Mumps, Rubella) vaccine. By the time of its introduction, the measles mortality rate had already
dropped significantly - from 13.3 in 100,000 in 1955 to
0.3 in 100,000. Historically, this disease, like similar
ones, has resulted in relatively high rates of complications and deaths among adolescents and young
adults, while doing no permanent or prolonged
damage to the pre-adolescent youth. The downgrading
of a disease such as measles from killer status to
'routine childhood disease' is indicative of the development of "herd" immunity in youngsters where the
disease, when contracted, follows a benign, self-limited
course. Measles is typically characterized by a skin
rash (pink spots) and a high fever. More serious
complications can include eye and ear inflammations,
pneumonia, and, in rare cases, encephalitis. Pneumonia
is the most common complication. In itself it too is
benign and self-limiting. Dr. Richard Moskowitz,
medical and homeopathic physician, tells us (<u>Dissent
in Medicine</u>, p. 148):

Ironically, what the measles vaccine has done is to reverse the historical or
evolutionary process to the extent that measles is once again a disease of
adolescents and young adults, with a correspondingly higher incidence of
pneumonia and other complications and a general tendency to be a more
serious and disabling disease than it usually is in younger children.

The measles vaccine is usually administered in a single
dose after one year of age.

MUMPS

Mumps is a viral disease, usually self-limiting, requiring no medical treatment. Once a child has contracted mumps, he will usually not develop the condition again, for acquisition of the disease typically
confers lifetime immunity on the recipient. Symptoms
of mumps include fever, headache, loss of appetite
and swelling of salivary glands.

Because of the benign nature of the disease, 16 of our 50 states do not require that the mumps portion of the MMR be given. Where required, one dose after the first birthday is usually given.

As with measles, Dr. Moskowitz tells us (<u>Dissent in Medicine</u>, p. 149) that mumps is now affecting an increasing number of adolescents and young adults. The chief complication, occurring in 30-40% of post-puberty males, is "acute epididymo-orchitis" which usually results in testicular atrophy on the affected side of the body. Also adversely affected are the pancreas and ovaries.

RUBELLA (GERMAN MEASLES)

The symptoms of rubella (3 day rash, fever, sore throat, mild 'cold') are at times so mild in young children as to go undiagnosed. In older children and in adults, however, the disease can produce more severe symptoms including arthritis and joint pain. The vaccine itself has also been known to cause such symptoms. The greatest risk posed by rubella is in exposure of a pregnant woman, for if she contracts the disease in her first trimester of pregnancy, damage to the developing embryo in the form of Congenital Rubella Syndrome (CRS) can result. The rubella out-break of 1964 resulted in a relatively high incidence of CRS, with an estimated 20,000 babies being affected. A mass "immunization" program followed in 1969. Rubella vaccine, like the measles vaccine, is generally administered in a single dose after 12 months of age.

Like measles and mumps, rubella is a relatively be-nign, self-limited disease of early childhood that poses little to no threat to young children. The MMR vac-cination however has transformed these diseases into more serious ones that are now affecting the very age groups (adolescent and young adult) most in need of protection from them.

DIPHTHERIA

Unlike measles, mumps and rubella, diphtheria and tetanus are serious diseases that can be fatal. Diphtheria vaccination is typically administered as part of the DPT inoculation (Diphtheria, Pertussis, Tetanus). Diphtheria and tetanus vaccines are not made from the living disease germs themselves, but rather from toxic substances associated with them. Tetanus and diphtheria 'toxoids' therefore seek to vaccinate not against the diseases themselves, but rather against the systemic effect of the original poisons. Both of these vaccines have been in use for a long time with a low incidence of reported problems stemming from their effects.

The necessity of the diphtheria vaccine is questionable however when we consider that the disease has nearly disappeared from the continent. The mortality rate had, in fact, *dropped by 50% prior to development of a vaccine* against diphtheria. And yet, today all 50 states require 3-5 doses, the last one usually given after the fourth birthday. Tetanus was likewise disappearing prior to the introduction of the vaccine. Both diseases furthermore are easily controlled by application of appropriate sanitation measures.

Evidence shows that the child who has not been vaccinated against diphtheria is no more susceptible to the disease than his 'fully immunized' counterpart. The Chicago Board of Health reported that in a 1969 outbreak of diphtheria, 25% of the children who contracted the disease had received all of the required vaccinations and another 12% had been given one or more doses of the vaccine, enough to show "serological evidence of full immunity" (Dr. Moskowitz, Dissent In Medicine, p.150). Another 18% had been partially vaccinated, making a total of 55% affected children who had been totally or partially 'immunized' and yet developed the disease.

TETANUS

Tetanus is technically not a childhood disease. It is a bacterial infection that can produce muscle spasms (spasms in the jaw = 'lockjaw') and neurological symptoms. The worldwide mortality rate is 30-50%, with the disease being particularly prevalent in tropical countries. 47 states require 1-5 inoculations of the tetanus virus, starting at age 2 months.

The tetanus vaccine, it has been found, may interfere with the immune reaction and has been linked with peripheral neuropathy, allergic reactions and laryngeal paralysis.

PERTUSSIS

Petussis, also known as whooping cough, is considered the most virulent of the childhood diseases. The predominant symptom of this potentially life threatening disease is a paroxysmal cough. A fever is also present. Frequency and severity of the disease had begun to decline significantly before the widespread use of the killed virus vaccine in 1957. In 1943, in fact, C.C. Dauer, epidemiologist, had remarked that, if mortality rate from pertussis were to decline at the then prevailing rate during the next 15 years, it would be 'extremely difficult' to statistically correlate its decline with use of the vaccine (developed in 1936). Today, however, 39 states require 3-5 doses of the injectable vaccine beginning at 2 months of age.

Pertussis has become the most controversial of the vaccinations due to claimed adverse effects which include central nervous system damage and hematological disturbances. The vaccine, while posing high risk, offers questionable immunity: According to the Center for Disease Control, of 759 cases of pertussis reported in infants in 1988, *49% had been fully immunized.*

POLIOMYELITIS

90% of persons infected with the poliomyelitis virus exhibit **no symptoms** and only 1-2% of the children infected exhibit 'classic' symptoms of the disease, meaning paralysis. Even at the zenith of the polio epidemic in this country in the 50s, 2/3 of the reported cases of polio were of the non-paralytic type, characterized by excess mucous, headaches, fever and 'aches and pains that come and go'. Polio vaccination is now required nationwide in 3-4 doses. It comes in two forms: a killed virus injection developed by Dr. Jonas Salk in 1955 and an orally administered live virus developed by Dr. Carl Sabin in 1960.

Aggressive vaccination programs are usually credited with virtually wiping out polio, with statistics reflecting a dramatic drop in the disease. In 1952 there were 57,879 reported cases and only 19 in 1971. That looks at first glance like a giant success attributable to the vaccines. Let's take a closer look:

When polio was in its heyday and running rampant, diagnosis of the disease could be made if the above listed non-paralytic symptoms persisted for a period of only **24 hours**. Look again at these symptoms: muscle aches, excess mucous, headaches and fever. Since there are 66 other diseases that produce the same symptoms and there was no test upon which to make a definitive, differential diagnosis, it is reasonable to believe that numerous people might have been diagnosed as having polio who may only have had a cold or some such benign ailment.

One huge factor in the rapid decline in the incidence of reported polio cases is attributable to a change in the required duration of symptoms for a condition to qualify as being diagnosed as polio. At the start of the 60s (when the Sabin vaccine was introduced), to be classified as 'polio', the above cold-like symptoms had to persist for **30 days** rather than 24 hours! As one can imagine, this resulted in a drastic drop in the number of reported cases. Also, in 1961, the incidence of a new disease, 'aseptic meningitis' rose in direct proportion to the decline in polio cases. It is interesting that the symptoms of aseptic meningitis are *exactly the same as the symptoms of polio* and, we are told (Anthony Robbins, <u>Fear Into Power</u> seminar, 1985), that both diseases are said to come from the *same virus*! In fact, Robbins cites statistics in a 1961-62 California medical journal that report zero polio cases, with a footnote stating: "all such cases now reported as *aseptic meningitis*"!

So, was it the vaccine or the re-defining of the criteria for diagnosing polio that accounted for the 'conquest' of the disease??

Dr. Moskowitz points out that a herd immunity had already begun to develop against polio prior to the introduction of the vaccine and that "immunity.. was already as close to being universal as it can ever be" (<u>Dissent in Medicine</u>, p. 152). Although Dr. Moskowitz states that the polio vaccine is "about as safe as any vaccine can be" (p. 153), Dr. Salk himself (who ironically became paralyzed) testified in front of Congress in 1980 that *95% of all polio cases* in the preceding 10 years had been *caused by the vaccine*!

HOW VACCINATIONS WORK

According to the 1986 <u>Red Book</u>, the pediatrician's reference book on the subject, "the goal [of vaccinations] is to mimic the natural infection by evoking an immunologic response which presents little or no risk to the recipient" (Richard Leviton, "Who Calls the Shots?" <u>Health Freedom News</u>, July/August, 1989). Many authorities seriously question both the effectiveness and the safety of the practice of vaccinating against disease. Objections are based in part on the arguments already mentioned - that disease rates were declining prior to the introduction of vaccines and the fact that many of the childhood diseases against which we routinely vaccinate are innocuous and self-limiting and therefore should be allowed to run their course. There is also the disturbing fact that many diseases have continued to appear in highly 'immunized' populations. Dr. Moskowitz postulates that vaccines offer only partial or temporary immunity, but observes that there is no way to tell how long such immunity will last. In addition to 'mimicking the natural infection', vaccines also produce their own sets of symptoms which, many experts tell us, may be more serious than the original disease. Dr. Robert Mendelsohn, M.D., practicing pediatrician for 25 years, as well as others in the field of holistic medicine, including Moskowitz, have expressed the opinion that vaccinations may have the long term effect of damaging the immune system. According to Mendelsohn, "the only proven characteristic of vaccines is their devastating adverse effects" (Richard Leviton, "Who Calls the Shots?" Health Freedom News, July/August, 1989.) Far from *enhancing* immunity, it is argued by Moskowitz that vaccinations may serve only to drive the disease deeper into the tissues, creating a *chronic* condition, wherein our response to the disease actually becomes progressively weaker. Vaccines typically involve the injection of viruses *directly into the bloodstream,* whereas in the normal course of the disease process, these organisms find their way into the body through one of the its orifices. Such ports-of-entry are equipped with filters to *protect* the bloodstream. By injecting the virus directly into the blood, we "give it free and immediate access to the major immune organs, without any obvious way of getting rid of it...[and thus] we have accomplished what the entire immune system seems to have evolved in order to prevent" (Moskowitz, Dissent in Medicine, p. 144). The result is *immunoSUPPRESSION,* the opposite of the claimed effect of the vaccination. Vaccinations result in the injected virus becoming permanently incorporated into the genetic material of the cell. Any antibodies produced by the body to combat that virus will therefore be directed against its own cells, resulting in autoimmune disease. Dr. Moskowitz concludes his argument by stating (Dissent in Medicine, p. 147):

If what I am saying turns out to be true, then what we have done by artificial immunizations is essentially to trade off our acute, epidemic diseases of the past century for the weaker and far less curable chronic diseases of the present, with their amortizable suffering and disability.

Often the association between the vaccination and the symptoms created by it is not made due to the time lapse between inoculation and the onset of symptoms, the parents lack of information re: the connection and the doctor's hesitancy in suggesting a causative link. Dr. Moskowitz suggests that homeopathy can be a valuable tool for *diagnosis* as well as treatment of vaccine-related disorders. He gives some brief case histories, describing how symptoms subsided rapidly after administration of a single dose of the appropriate homeopathic dilution of the virus.

BUBBLE, BUBBLE, TOIL AND TROUBLE

As of 1988, there were 19 licensed vaccines in this country, including the 7 already described. These vaccines contain either a live or killed infectious agent, usually a virus or bacteria, as well as sterile water (used as a suspending agent), preservatives (including formaldehyde and mercury derivatives), stabilizers, antibiotics and adjuvants (aluminum phosphate). Hannah Allen (Don't Get Stuck, p. 22) tells us that the materials from which the "vaccines, serums and biologicals" are produced include:

1) ROTTEN HORSE BLOOD (FOR DIPHTHERIA TOXIN AND ANTITOXIN)
2) MACERATED CANCEROUS BREASTS
3) SWEEPINGS FROM VACUUM CLEANERS (FOR ASTHMA AND HAY FEVER)
4) PUS FROM SORES OF DISEASED ANIMALS
5) METALLIC POISONS
6) POWDERED INSECTS
7) MUCOUS FROM THE THROATS OF CHILDREN WITH COLDS AND WHOOPING COUGH
8) DECOMPOSED FECAL MATTER FROM TYPHOID PATIENTS

9) SEWAGE
10) URINE
11) FECAL MATTER
12) GARBAGE
13) DISHWATER

Is it really scientific or even rational to believe that having the above items injected into our bloodstream will confer immunity from disease?? It may not be rational, but it **is** big business in this country and worldwide and we might therefore suspect vested interest, rather than disease prevention, as a prime motivating factor in promotion of vaccinations.

It is not surprising, in view of the above list, to note that vaccinations have actually been linked with development of such virulent diseases as Epstein-Barr Virus (EBV) and AIDS. As reported by Richard Leviton in his "Who Calls the Shots?" article in the July/August 1989 issue of Health Freedom News, the time table looks something like this:

1985: A SCIENTIST AT HARVARD'S SCHOOL OF PUBLIC HEALTH REVEALED THAT AN AIDS TYPE VIRUS (STLV-3) HAS BEEN FOUND IN THE AFRICAN GREEN MONKEY WHOSE KIDNEY CELLS WERE USED TO CULTURE ORAL POLIO VIRUS.

1987: THE LONDON TIMES REPORTED THAT THE PREVALENCE OF SMALLPOX VACCINATIONS OVER 13 YEARS IN 7 AFRICAN NATIONS TRIGGERED THE AIDS VIRUS OUTBREAK THERE.

1988: THE BRITISH MEDICAL JOURNAL, MEDICAL HYPOTHESIS, IN A STUDY OF 200 PATIENTS WITH CHRONIC EBV, REPORTED IT WAS CAUSED BY THE LIVE RUBELLA VIRUS FOUND IN THE VACCINE.

THE HISTORICAL PERSPECTIVE

Preventive vaccination was first promoted in 1796 by Dr. Edward Jenner of England who developed a cowpox vaccination against smallpox. Use of his vaccine led to massive outbreaks of the disease and it was therefore banned by 1837.

Vaccinations are no longer compulsory in England, West Germany of Sweden, and it's reported that since the decline in pertussis immunizations, hospitalizations and death rates from the disease have fallen in England.

Vaccinations were made non-compulsory in England due largely to the findings of Professor Alfred Russel Wallace, Anthony Robbins tells us (Fear Into Power seminar, 1985). Dr. Wallace was asked by Encyclopedia Brittanica to write an article about how smallpox was wiped out by vaccinations. In his investigations, Robbins tells us, Dr. Wallace found that in countries where the vaccine was introduced, smallpox multiplied *15 times and that 65-70% of the people who contracted the disease had been vaccinated against it.* He wrote up these findings in a chapter called "The Pursuit of Evil", part of a larger volume entitled The Wonderful Century. The interesting thing, Robbins states, is that this chapter just happens to have been eliminated from all copies of this book found in the U.S., except one: The one complete volume is housed at Yale University. It may not be checked out, but can be read only on the premises in a locked room! Do you get the impression that information is being withheld on the subject?? As regards smallpox, it is also an interesting, little-known fact that Dr. Charles A.R. Campbell, who was recommended for the Nobel Prize around the turn of the century, discovered that the disease was caused by the bite of a blood-sucking insect, the bedbug, that it was not infectious nor contagious and that vaccinations do not prevent it.

THE LEGAL PERSPECTIVE

Prior to 1988, there was no nationwide mandated reporting system requiring reports to be filed on adverse reactions to vaccinations. Therefore, we have no accurate data on the subject. As things stand now, it is unknown how many of the 67,000 infants vaccinated weekly in the U.S. may be suffering from adverse reactions. Barbara Fisher, co-author of DPT: A Shot in the Dark and mother of a DPT vaccine injured child founded D.P.T. (Dissatisfied Parents Together) in 1982 for the purpose of enhancing public awareness and initiating legislative action. In their book, she and co-author, Harris Coulter estimate as many as 943 deaths and 11,666 cases of long term damage from DPT vaccinations.

In his book, Dangers of Compulsory Immunizations: How to Avoid them Legally, attorney Tom Finn cites the legal aspects, precedents and strategies of avoid-ance of vaccinations. He tells us that the courts have proclaimed that consumers must be adequately warned of the dangers of vaccines by the drug manufacturers and that failure to give such warning opens them up to liability for injuries. He adds an interesting perspec-tive on that ruling (p. 13):

IT SEEMS INCONSISTENT TO REQUIRE THE MANUFACTURER TO WARN THE CONSUMER OF THE POTENTIAL DANGERS CON-NECTED WITH THE VACCINE'S USE AND THEN COMPEL AN INDIVIDUAL TO BE INJECTED AGAINST THEIR WILL. IF THE CONSUMER IS NOT ALLOWED TO MAKE THIS CHOICE BECAUSE OF A COMPULSORY IMMUNIZATION STATUTE, THEN THE GOVERNMENT IS EXPOSING ITSELF TO LIABILITY FOR ANY RE-SULTING INJURIES EITHER UNDER THE THEORY THAT THEY'RE FORCING THE INOCULATION ON THE PARTY OR UNDER THE THEORY THAT THE GOVERNMENT HAS WARRANTED THAT THE DRUG IS SAFE. IT COULD BE ARGUED THAT THE GOVERN-MENT HAS GIVEN ITS SEAL OF APPROVAL TO THE VACCINATION BY COMPELLING INDIVIDUALS UNDER PENALTY OF LAW TO BE VACCINATED.

While all states require vaccinations as a pre-requisite to public school admission, exemptions may be granted for medical reasons in all 50 states. Religious exemp-tions are allowed in all states except West Virginia and Mississippi and philosophical exemptions may now be granted in 22 states. These exemptions offer a way out for parents choosing not to expose their children to the potential dangers of compulsory vaccinations.

The three major manufacturers of vaccines - American Cyanamide, Lederle and Wyeth - have had hundreds of lawsuits filed against them since 1984. Many have been settled out of court, with a ban on publicity. Of those that have gone to court, the majority of rulings have been in favor of the manufacturers. In 1987 the U.S. Department of Justice intervened as a 'friend of the court' in support of Wyeth Laboratory, thus overturning a $2.1 million damage decision that had been rendered in favor of a DPT injured child. Several large monetary settlements have been awarded to injured parties, including $15 million (Graham vs. Wyeth, 1987) to a child who became retarded after his first DPT shot.

In 6/88 Congress appropriated $320 million to compensate parents of vaccine-damaged or killed children prior to 10/88. Parents can file a law suit against the drug company involved or apply for federal compensation at a fixed rate in accordance with the National Childhood Vaccine Injury Act up through January 31, 1991.

More information on the dangers associated with vaccinations is available through The Vaccine Research Institute, P.O. Box 4182, Northbrook, Illinois 60065. They publish a list of reference articles available for $3.00.

The theory that vaccinations can confer immunity against disease is an outgrowth of the theory that germs cause disease which was explored in chapter 2. If, as suggested, autotoxemia is instead the root cause of disease because it creates a cellular environment conducive to the proliferation of germs, then the entire theoretical framework supporting vaccinations (and the whole of the medical model) proves unsound. And, it can be readily seen how the vaccines add to the body's toxic burden, thus *reducing immunity*, rather than enhancing it.

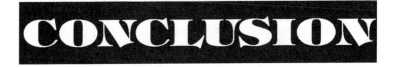
CONCLUSION

It is hoped that the information in this book has prompted the reader to reassess some basic assumptions about disease causation and health maintenance. In preceding pages we have challenged the validity of such traditional beliefs as:

- GERMS CAUSE DISEASE
- VACCINATIONS PREVENT DISEASE
- FLUORIDE PREVENTS TOOTH DECAY
- DAIRY PRODUCTS ARE THE BEST SOURCE OF CALCIUM
- EXTREMELY LOW ELECTRICAL FREQUENCIES ARE HARMLESS
- SUNLIGHT CAUSES CANCER
- EATING MEAT MAKES US STRONG
- PASTEURIZATION ASSURES CLEANLINESS OF MILK
- DENTAL AMALGAMS ARE PERFECTLY SAFE
- WE SHOULD EAT FROM EACH OF THE 4 FOOD GROUPS DAILY

In the forefront of today's health revolution are those daring to challenge the above premises and seeking alternatives to medical treatment of disease.

There is dissent even within the 'holistic movement', for health care alternatives run the gamut from the strict vegetarian/raw-food-only/no supplements hygienist approach through the philosophy that advocates megadoses of isolated nutrients and chemical compounds. In between these extremes we find the macrobiotic approach which emphasizes balance and cooks everything. We believe there is some degree of merit in all of these approaches. Macrobiotics, with its emphasis upon whole grains and sea vegetables, provides us with an abundant source of minerals and B vitamins so deficient in the SAD. The hygienist emphasis on raw foods and proper food combining conserves energy by providing food enzymes and allowing energy previously used for digestion to be redirected into regeneration. Megavitamin therapy, too, can have a place, as a temporary replacement for drug therapy to alleviate symptoms until balance can be restored in the body through dietary control.

It is imperative that the various alternative philosophies and modalities realize and emphasize their common bonds rather than their differences, for there are elements within the medical establishment that have launched an all-out smear campaign against what they view as their competition. In his well documented book, The Great Medical Monopoly Wars, P.J. Lisa reveals that for more than three decades the AMA and its allies have been secretly conspiring to destroy their competitors in the alternative health care fields. Monies from vested interests have financed campaigns against 'health fraud' and 'quacks' purportedly aimed at 'protecting' the public. From whom are they protecting us? from their competition! What is apparent is that their primary goal is maintaining their medical monopoly, not safeguarding our health. Division within the holistic sector can only profit those who seek to discredit natural healing and its practitioners.

We envision a time, at the height of the New Age, when allopathic medicine, with its toxic drugs and invasive surgical procedures, falls into virtual disuse, when the giant pharmaceutical interests disintegrate for lack of support. Thomas Edison once said:

The doctor of the furure will give no medicine but will interest his patients in the care of the human frame, in diet, and in the cause and prevention of disease.

Edison's future vision is dawning in today's holistic health movement. And, interestingly, the Aquarian air element, electricity, for which he is so well known, is destined to play a key role as a major healing modality in the future.

BOOK ORDER FORM

Please send _____ copy (copies) of <u>The Book of Health</u> to:

Name (please print) _____

Street Address or P.O. _____

City, State, Zip _____

QUANTITY DISCOUNTS AVAILABLE

Number of Copies	Price Per Copy
1	$12.95
2-3	$11.95
4-5	$10.95
5 or more	$9.95

ADD POSTAGE AND HANDLING

1-2 books	$2.00
3-4 books	$4.00
5 books or more	$5.00

Florida residents add 6% sales tax.

Please send this order form with a check or money order to:

Susan Stockton
329 North 13th Street
Haines City, FL 33844

Inquiries regarding workshop presentations welcomed.

BIBLIOGRAPHY

BOOKS

Abrahamson, E.M., M.D. and A.W. Pezet. Body, Mind and Sugar. New York: Avon Books, 1951.

Aihara, Herman. Acid and Alkaline. Oroville, California: George Oshawa Macrobiotic Foundation, 1986.

Airola, Paavo PhD., N.D. How to Get Well. Phoenix, Arizona: Health Plus Publishers, 1974.

Allen, Hannah. Don't Get Stuck. Oldsmar, Florida: Natural Hygiene Press, 1985.

Banik, Allen E., Dr. The Choice is Clear. Raytown, Missouri: Acres U.S.A., 1975.

Becker, Robert O., M.D. and Gary Selden. The Body Electric. New York: Quill, 1985.

Bird, Christopher. The Life and Trials of Gaston Naessens, The Galileo of the Microscope, St. Lambert, Québec, Canada: Les Presses de l'Université de la Personne Inc., 1990.

Bliznakov, Emile G., M.D. and Gerald L. Hunt. The Miracle Nutrient Coenzyme Q 10. New York: Bantam Books, 1987.

Burroughs, Stanley. The Master Cleanser. Auburn, California: Stanley Burroughs, 1976.

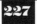

Cousens, Gabriel, M.D. Spiritual Nutrition and the Rainbow Diet. Boulder, Colorado: Cassandra Press, 1986.

Cousins, Norman. Anatomy of an Illness. New York: Bantam Books, 1979.

Davis, Adelle. Let's Eat Right to Keep Fit. New York: Harcourt, Brace, Jovanovich, Inc., 1970.

Diamond, Harvey and Marilyn. Fit for Life. New York: Warner Books, 1987.

Diamond, John, M.D. Your Body Doesn't Lie. New York: Warner Books, 1979.

Donsbach, Kurt W., PhD., D.Sc., N.D., D.C. Dr. Donsbach Tells You What You Always Wanted to Know About Water. Huntington Beach, California: The International Institute of Natural Health Sciences, 1981.

Dufty, William. Sugar Blues. Denver, Colorado: Nutri-Books Corporation, 1975.

Finn, Tom, Attorney. Dangers of Compulsory Immunizations. How to Legally Avoid Them. New Port Richey, Florida: Fitness Press, 1983.

Guyton, Arthur C., M.D. Textbook of Medical Physiology. 6th edition, W.B. Saunders Co., 1981.

Hoffman, Jay, PhD. What's Wrong with Meat? Valley Center, California: Professional Press Publishing Association, 1985.

Honorof, Ida and E. McBean. Vaccinations The Silent Killer. A Clear and Present Danger. Sherman Oaks, California: Honor Publications, 1977.

Howell, Dr. Edward. Enzyme Nutrition. The Food Enzyme Concept. Wayne, New Jersey: Avery Publishing Group, 1985.

Hume, Elizabeth Douglas. Béchamp or Pasteur? A Lost Chapter in the History of Biology, London: The C.W. Daniel Company, reprinted 1989 by Health Research, Mokelumne Hill, CA.

James, Walene. Immunization: The Reality Behind the Myth. New York: Bergin and Garvey, 1988.
Jensen, Bernard. Nature Has a Remedy. Escondido, California: Dr. Bernard Jensen, 1978.

Jensen, Dr. Bernard, D.C. Tissue Cleansing Through Bowel Management. Escondido, California: Bernard Jensen, 1981.

Kervran, Louis. Biological Transmutations. Woodstock, New York: Beekman Publishers, Inc., 1980.

Kime, Zane R., M.D.. M.S. Sunlight. Penryn, California: World Health Publications, 1980.

Kirschmann, John D. with Lavon J. Dunne. Nutrition Almanac. New York: McGraw-Hill Company, Nutrition Search, Inc., 1973.

Kroeger, Hanna, MsD., Rev. Old Time Remedies for Modern Ailments. Rev. Hanna Kroeger, MsD., 1971.

Kushi, Michio and Aveline. Macrobiotic Diet. Tokyo, New York: Japan Publications, 1985.

Lisa, P.J. The Great Medical Monopoly Wars. Huntington Beach, California: International Institute of Natural Health Sciences, Inc., 1986.

Lynes, Barry with John Crane. The Cancer Cure that Worked. Toronto, Canada: Marcus Books, 1987.

Manthei, Joseph C., D.C. Health Through Diet. Drumore, Pennsylvania: More Excellent Ways Ministries, 1979.

Mendelsohn, Robert S., M.D., et al. Dissent in Medicine. Nine Doctors Speak Out. Chicago, Illinois: Contemporary Books, Inc., 1985.

Mindell, Earl. Unsafe at Any Meal. New York: Warner Books, 1987.

McDougall, John A., M.D. The McDougall Plan. Piscataway, New Jersey: New Century Publishers, Inc., 1983.

Oldfield, Harry and Roger Coghill. The Dark Side of the Brain. Longmead, Shaftesbury, Dorset, England: Element Books, 1988.

Ott, John N. Health and Light. New York: Pocket Books, 1973.

Parham, Vistara. What's Wrong With Eating Meat? Denver, Colorado: PCAP Publications, 1979.

Passwater, Richard A., Ph.D. and Elmer M. Cranton, M.D. Trace Elements, Hair Analysis and Nutrition. Keats Publishing, 1983.

Philpott, William H., M.D. and Dwight K. Kalita, PhD. Brain Allergies. New Canaan, Connecticut: Keats Publishing, Inc., 1980.

Reckeweg, Dr. Hans Heinrich, Homotoxicology. Albuquerque, New Mexico: Menaco Publishing Co., Inc. 1984.

Reilly, Harold J., D.Ph.T., D.S. and Ruth Hagy Brod. The Edgar Cayce Handbook for Health Through Drugless Therapy. New York: McMillan Publishing Company, 1975.

Samuels, Mike, M.D. and Hal Bennett. The Well Body Book. New York: Random House/Bookworks, 1973.

Schauss, Alexander, M.A. Diet, Crime and Delin-quency. Berkeley, California: Parker House, 1981.

Tobe, John H. Hydrogenation - America's Deadliest Killer. St. Catharines, Ontario: Modern Publications Reg'd, 1962.

Walker, N.W., D.Sc. Fresh Vegetable and Fruit Juices. Phoenix, Arizona: O'Sullivan, Woodside and Company, 1936.

Webb, Tony, et. al. Food Irradiation: Who Wants It? Rochester, Vermont: Thorsons Publishers, Inc., 1987.

Weinberger, Stanley. Colon Health - Pathway to Health.

West, Samuel C., D.N., N.D. The Golden Seven Plus One. Orem, Utah: Samuel Publishing Company, 1981.

Williams, Dr. Roger, J. Nutrition Against Disease. New York: Bantam Books, 1973.

Yao, George, T.F. Pulsor Miracle of Microcrystals. A Treatise on Energy Balancing. Newport Beach, California: Gyro Industries, 1986.

Yiamouyiannis, Dr. John. Fluoride The Aging Factor. Delaware, Ohio: Health Action Press, 1986.

Ziff, Sam. Silver Dental Fillings. The Toxic Time Bomb. new York: Aurora Press, 1984.

Ziff, Sam and Michael F. Ziff, D.D.S. The Hazards of Silver/Mercury Dental Fillings. Orlando, Florida: Bio-Probe, Inc. 1985.

_____. Facts You Should Know About Water Fluoridation. Mokelumne Hill, California: Health Research.

MAGAZINES AND NEWSLETTERS

Becker, Robert O., M.D. "Brain Pollution". Psychology Today. February, 1979.

Bird, Christopher. "Seaponics and Sonic Bloom — or Sound and Nutrients". Acres U.S.A. June, 1985.

Biser, Sam and Loren. "How Increasing Your Energy Affects Your Emotions, Your Personality and Your Sex Life". The Healthview Newsletter (#27-29). December, 1981.

Brodeur, Paul. "Annals of Radiation." New Yorker. July 9, 1990.

Bruce, Gene. "The Myth of Vegetarian B12." East/West Journal. May, 1988.

Chatsworth, Colin and Loren. "The Great Vitamin C Debate." The Healthview Special Report (newsletter). Charlottesville, Virginia: Colin and Loren Chatsworth. 1985.

Considine, Harvey. "Homogenized Milk, Not Cholesterol Real Villian of Heart Disease." Dairy Goat Journal. May, 1979. (from Acres USA, 8/78 issue).

Cowley, Geoffrey. "An Electromagnetic Storm". Newsweek. July, 10, 1989.

Goldhamer, Alan, D.C. "Do You Really Need Vitamin Supplements?" Health Science. November/December, 1989.

Grauerholz, Dr. John. "The Nobel fakery of Linus Pauling". EIR. August 28, 1984.

Fels, Harriet. "Fluoridation: Health Measure or Hoax?" East/West Journal. October, 1989.

Kotzsch, Ronald. "Bring the Sun Indoors." East/West Journal. March, 1989.

Leviton, Richard. "Who Calls the Shots?" Health Freedom News. July/August, 1989.

London, Wayne P. "Full Spectrum Classroom Light and Sickness in Pupils." The Lancet, volume II. November 21, 1987.

Moore, William H. "Mercurophilia in American Health Care". Wellness Lifestyle. May, 1990.

Ponte, Lowell. "The Menace of Electric Smog." Reader's Digest. January, 1980.

Scala, James, M.D. "EPA Update, Part I: Research Continues". Alive.

_____. "Everything You Always Wanted to Know About Calcium". Long Beach, California: Nature's Plus, 1986.

Williams, Dr. David G. Alternatives. (Vol. 3, No. 19). January, 1991.

Wurtman, Richard J. "The Effects of Light on the Human Body." The Scientific American. July, 1975.

TAPES

Irons V.E. "Detoxify: Enzyme Activity and Rejuvenation", National Health Federation Convention lecture, 1983.

Pritikin, Nathan. "Lipotoxemia: Nutrition and Degenerative Disease". Santa Monica, California: Pritikin Longevity Center, 1980.

Puharich, Andrija, M.D., LL.D. "The Final Solution to the ELF Problem."

Robbins, Anthony. "Ten Keys to Health" from 'Fear Into Power' and 'Nutrition' seminar, April, 1985.

LECTURE TRANSCRIPT

Morrell, Dr. Franz. "The Bio-Electronic Method of Prof. Vincent" from O.I.C.S. Alumni Association's German Electro-Acupuncture week in July, 1982 at El Rancho Inn, Millbrae, California.